Getting Cracked

Preparing for open heart surgery
2nd Edition

Getting Cracked

Preparing for open heart surgery
2nd Edition

Written By:
Jon Frazier

Cover Art By:
Cash Wheeler

In memory of Maxie, her love for others was the purest religion...

Chapter 1

Where Do We Begin?

Every year, approximately half a million people have open-heart surgery in the United States, according to Antony Chu, MD, of the Warren Alpert Medical School of Brown University. This number appears less drastic when you realize that the Centers for Disease Control have listed heart disease as the leading cause of death among both males and females for many years. This single statistic might highlight why you are turning the pages of this book at this very moment.

This book won't be a love story between a vampire and a human girl or some type of fast-paced thriller. Possibly, you could be a colleague of mine curious to know if I can string two words together coherently, or my mother. Most likely you are one of the people who are either having open-heart surgery or know someone who is going to have open-heart surgery. If that is what brought you to this point, then you have taken a step in the right direction toward building up a knowledge base to help you prepare for a life-changing event.

This is my story. Some parts of the story might be unique to me, while others might be similar to everyone else who has ever had open-heart surgery. My hope in writing this book is that you might be able to learn a little something about the surgery. There is a chance you might learn even more than you would like. Chances are you could have a laugh at my expense along the way. This story will cover a lot of the gory details of the process of correcting a heart problem with surgery.

I am certain that some people will find this book to be too graphic with the information included, while others will think it isn't detailed enough. There are usually a group of scary movie junkies in every crowd. Perhaps the rest of the surgery crowd will shrug this information off as common knowledge and tell their friends they already knew everything they read anyway.

Hopefully, you know which of those categories you fall into, so we can jump right into the thick of it. I can't possibly discuss in detail the differences in every procedure because this isn't an introductory course to a cardiac fellowship, and I am way too lazy for that anyway. If you do have some specific questions about the type of procedure you are having, be warned that the internet can be your best friend and your worst enemy at the same time. Never be afraid to talk to your doctor if you feel like you need more details on what the specifics of your surgery will be.

The first thing we need to touch on will be how recently medical professionals started doing heart surgery. If you haven't already looked it up, take a moment to consider how long surgeons have been operating on people's hearts. How long has the medical community been working to smooth the creases out of heart surgery? Thirty years, maybe forty? Or are you the type of person who likes a long shot and said a hundred years? Do you think doctors started repairing hearts before or after the great depression?

Do you find it hard to believe that the first credited heart surgery was performed over one hundred and twenty years ago in Chicago, Illinois? According to Columbia Surgery's website, the first successful heart surgery occurred in 1893 by Dr. Daniel Hale Williams.

The son of a barber who also founded an integrated teaching hospital, was the first to successfully repair a damaged left internal mammary artery. The doctor then managed to hand-sew the pericardium through an incision between the patient's ribs. Dr. Williams suspected a heart injury when the patient started going into shock after a stabbing. With limited time and a pioneering spirit, he made repairs that were unheard of at the time through just a crack of space.

Dr. Williams recognized a problem, repaired it, and saved James Cornish's life that night. Mr. Cornish would walk out of that hospital in Chicago after fifty-one days. It is an interesting story that everyone should consider.

Yet the real surprise that should spring to mind is the fact that heart surgery in some form has been happening a lot longer than you have been alive. While the techniques have evolved over time, increasing efficiency and safety for patients, the surgery itself predates Coca-Cola. That company, an institution of American cold refreshments, wouldn't sell its first bottle until the following year.

It is true that James Cornish had a stab wound repaired and was able to go home in less than two months. While this won't be the same type of open-heart procedure this book details, it is still wildly impressive that this repair was done successfully so many years ago.

It is also true that I was able to have my aorta replaced with a synthetic graft and leave for my own home in five days time. I know that was a spoiler. There could have been an entire group of readers believing I was writing this from beyond the grave. If that was you, I am sorry I ruined it for you. No refunds.

This book will aim to be a personal how-to guide to mentally and physically prepare for your open-heart procedure. I will touch on the aspects of preparing for a surgery that were new to me on a personal level, even though I spend most of my professional days in the operating room as a Certified Registered Nurse Anesthetist (CRNA). Most of all, it will be my story. The first thing I can encourage people to do from the very beginning of this process is to document your personal story. I truly hope you can enjoy my story because writing it down helped me deal with some of the mentally taxing portions of the healing process.

As we begin this journey together, remember some important facts as you are reading. I made it. This book will not be built up for a big reveal at the end. It is not ghost-written, pun intended. It is okay to laugh. I want you to laugh at me, and when the time is right, maybe even laugh at yourself. Whoever said laughter is the best medicine obviously didn't need open-heart surgery. But laughter is still a good alternative to feeling better in a bad situation. Not as good as drugs, but still better than depression. Whether or not you want to prepare yourself or ignore the date altogether, your surgery *will* happen.

Keep those things in mind as we start getting you ready for your big day in the operating room.

Make notes, highlight stuff, and buy ten more copies for your closest friends. Whatever makes you happy. Stop by my page on Instagram at *"gettingcrackedthebook"* with pictures of me in all my glory throughout the process so you can visualize what it is I am talking about as well. That account will take you on a visual journey from the preoperative me, all the way through the procedure, and you can even see what my incisions look like now. You can drop me a line on the site as well if you have additional questions like how many copies is too many copies? Just have fun and let's get informed.

Chapter 2
A Little History

As I sit here writing this, months into my postoperative period and not fully recovered from my surgery, I guess you might be wondering what got me to this point. I am only forty-four years old, which may seem a little young to be having open-heart surgery. It happens. Nobody assumes they are going to be hitting the grind at work, ramping up their career, and watching their children grow up when suddenly they need to take a pause and head to the hospital for a life-changing event. Of course, no one plans to get in a car wreck either. It just kind of happens. Remember that. For so many of these types of surgeries, people wonder what they could have done to prevent it. Many times, the answer is nothing.

As I mentioned, despite my graying hair that keeps receding slowly to the back of my head, I am still a younger guy. Forty-four is the new forty, or something to that nature. My cardiologist says I am overweight based on my body mass index, which is simply the calculation of weight mixed with height. You can find average ranges on numerous web pages if you are curious about where you might fall. A good place to start might be the cdc.gov website.

Specifically, the body mass index (BMI) is defined as a person's mass (weight in kilograms) divided by their height in meters squared. The American version of that calculation is 703 x weight (lbs)/ [height (in)]^2 for those who refuse to consider the metric system. When someone says, "I am a little short for my weight," it is a subtle BMI joke. A BMI of 25 or greater is designated as overweight. And BMI is just like any other risk factor□ the farther away from normal you deviate, the higher your risk increases for other issues.

However, my BMI doesn't even consider how active I am! Just to clarify, I am not very active at all. I am an average height, average weight white guy who has always been viewed as relatively in shape. I had no medical history that made me sit up and say, "I need to make some changes." At least I have never said that in regards to my health. As we get older, our activity levels will normally diminish. The leading cause of being overweight for me was a raging case of apathy. No health issue kept me from exercising, just sheer laziness on my part. In spite of that laziness, I was still able to manage a somewhat slimmer physique, even if the numbers said otherwise. My only saving grace is the fact that I log a lot of steps at work every day.

At this point, I sound like an uninteresting Dr. Seuss character...

I am not fat,
I am not small,
I am not short,
I am not tall...

It is all of these things that make this book correlate to ordinary people as well as those who have a glaring health deficit that screams, "I need heart surgery!" Heart surgery can happen to anyone at any time. It does not discriminate. Remember this fact if you are a family member learning for the first time that someone you know needs an operation. Very often, this is not the consequence of a poor lifestyle choice.

As I mentioned, I work in the healthcare field as a nurse anesthetist. That just means that I spend most of my days in an operating room delivering anesthesia to people having surgery. The majority of my time, I am working with people who are extremely knowledgeable about health issues. This fact might clear up some confusion later when I reference having a conversation with someone at work. It's not the same as when Bob from the construction site, who drinks a twelve-pack a day and is seventy pounds overweight, says his knee problems are genetic because his mother was Irish. I am not saying Bob is wrong. He is, but I'm not saying it. I am only saying that the people I talk to at work about health problems are certified experts in the field, not just random strangers who have done an internet search.

Here I was, just having a normal day at work. I was chatting about life and the moves throughout several careers that had brought my family and I to the area several years earlier. A surgeon asked me to clarify something I had mentioned about my father. I had casually referenced that he had passed away some years earlier from a heart attack. We will later refer to this as a heart event instead of a heart attack because that will be more honest in reality. Since there was no autopsy done, we do not know the specifics of what happened with his passing other than the fact it had to do with his heart.

On the night of my father's untimely death, he was sitting in his recliner as he had done countless times before. He had retired from years of working in a paper mill, spending the bulk of his workday fairly inactive sitting at a computer console. My father was affectionately known as Big John by those closest to him. It was never meant to be an insult, but used because his habitus earned it.

He was a big man. Big John might have had twiggy legs, but he was tall with a robust midsection. The man was overweight in the real sense and was still a smoker at the time of his passing. Big John had a history of multiple transient ischemic attacks (TIA) in the past, which is similar to a mini-stroke for lack of a better term. This was a man who enjoyed every facet of his life, and it showed a bit in his physique.

The short version is that he had a pain in his chest, mentioned it to my mother, and then tried to play it off by asking her to go get a pizza instead of calling 911. Just to clarify, my mother did not leave for the pizza. A few moments later, my father grabbed his chest and hit the floor. He was gone in minutes. Paramedics would attempt to revive him, but my father never regained consciousness. Just like that, he was gone from our lives forever.

That was the story of my father. The question on everyone's mind was what I had changed in my own life with a heart history in my family like that? How did it affect my lifestyle, exercise, or eating? These were all excellent questions. Alas, I did not give an excellent answer. My answer was nothing. No change in diet or exercise. I hadn't done much of anything in the way of altering my lifestyle to accommodate for a family history of heart issues. But I was young and in decent shape, so why would I worry?

The next question asked of me was who I was seeing as my cardiologist. I felt bad that this guy was a surgeon and had such a hard time listening. I was not seeing anyone, because I was healthy. There had not been any problems at all, except for a little bit of chest pain when I was lifting something heavy a few years back. I guess there were also some smaller pains at other times, but I was positive those were flukes.

There are moments in your life that remain as crystal clear as when they happened for months or even years after they occur. The birth of a child, the death of a loved one, and the soul-sucking stare of a surgeon that pierces through time and space when he tells you he is writing an order for blood work today. Blood work that you will be getting done immediately.

Have you ever been casually carrying on a conversation, convinced you weren't the dumbest person in the room only to find out that everyone else assumed you must have a learning disability as soon as you opened your mouth? It had been a while for me, so I decided to see if both feet would fit in my mouth. I can read the health history of a patient and know the best course of action to keep them safe in the operating room with ease. Yet when it came to my own health, and recommendations that might inconvenience me, I had blinders on. This fact alone makes me relatable to most people in the general population. How many people have truly taken care of their health throughout their life? It's tough to eat healthy and exercise can be a real pain to fit into a busy schedule.

Seriously, I thought this surgeon was a pretty chill guy. Oddly enough, when I mentioned I had not had any heart issues except some chest pain, he instantly became perplexed at how I had gotten so far in my career while ignoring some fairly obvious signs of distress. I liked this surgeon a lot, so I figured it was easier to have a blood draw than to argue with him. And it was. I had my blood drawn the next day and opened the results with him later. In retrospect, I should have opened those lab results alone, because no one likes to hear the phrase "I told you so."

All my lab results were off. My lipid panel looked like I was a guy who never watched what he ate and rarely exercised. I wonder why?

A lipid panel is a blood test that evaluates the levels of lipids, which are nothing more than the fats used as a source of energy by your body. Lipids include cholesterol, triglycerides, high-density lipoprotein (HDL), and low-density lipoprotein (LDL).

High cholesterol is an easy fix. It was as simple as a prescription for medication to get my labs in order. A common medication to help with cholesterol is a statin. Perhaps you have already started treatment with this type of drug as well. During a recheck after being on medication for a bit, my labs looked fine. Fixing my cholesterol was as simple as taking a single pill a day. Of course, now I am taking that pill for the rest of my life.

This was another "aha" moment that unfortunately for me didn't resonate quite loudly enough. You would think that possibly a man with three kids, a wife, and a mound of debt would take better care of himself. For all the ladies reading this, I am going to let you in on a little secret about men. We are pretty dumb when it comes to admitting that we are getting older. I know what you're thinking. "I'll take obvious facts about men for $500, Alex."

Because I now have a tiny glimpse into the truth that I was aging, I had to use my huge brain to determine if that single test was good enough for me and my family. Ultimately, I admitted to myself that there was a possibility my health was not where it needed to be. Months later, I saw another guy I liked at work who is a cardiologist, and I asked if he would schedule me for an office visit. We discussed my history and the bloodwork, and he was in agreement that I should be seeing a cardiologist as a precautionary measure.

This is a luxury I have in my profession, and I am well aware that it is not something most people will share with me. As you are reading this, I hope you realize that I had every resource at my disposal without having to worry about referrals or secretaries or insurance. Yet I still waited, subconsciously knowing that I was putting myself and my family at risk for nothing more than foolish pride. I refer to this as M&M disorder. This is where my brain works normally for others, but when it has to make sound decisions for me it has a thick candy shell.

In your mind, perhaps you are calculating how fast I was able to get all of this done. In all honesty, it was eighteen months of me delaying and being lazy before I finally made the appointment to do what I was supposed to do. Never underestimate a man's apathy when it could affect his bad eating habits and indifferent attitude toward exercise. I can only hope that the people who are making a plan at this point were more aggressive with their health plan than I was at the time.

After such a long wait, I saw my cardiologist, had an electrocardiogram (ECG), and everything looked normal. There were no funny heart rhythms, and no previous infarcts were noted.

An ECG is a medical test that can detect cardiac abnormalities by measuring the electrical activity generated by the heart as it contracts, using a series of electrodes placed on the chest and extremities.

Although my heart rhythm was normal, it did not mean this cardiologist gave me a lollipop and sent me on my way. His advice to me was to lose some weight, get some exercise, and have a great life. Oh, by the way, maybe it would be a good idea at my age to grab a stress echo and make sure there are no problems with my heart when it is beating at a significantly higher rate than when resting. Easy peasy, lemon squeezy.

This exam can be called a stress test, stress echocardiography test, or simply a stress echo. This is the test where they hook you up to a stack of electrodes, put you on a treadmill, and start turning it up until your heart beats faster than normal to see how it responds before, during, and after the stress is applied. The women who administered my test had a great sense of humor because they just laughed and laughed when I told them I was in pretty good shape.

The common steps of a stress test using a treadmill:

1. The patient is hooked up to the device that monitors the heart with electrodes and wires that will be there for the duration of the time on the treadmill.
2. A blood pressure cuff is wrapped around the upper part of one arm to monitor the different blood pressures before, during, and after the exam.
3. The patient will then stand on the treadmill.
4. The treadmill starts to move, and the patient walks slowly at first, answering questions about fatigue and breathing.
5. The treadmill speed will begin to gradually increase.
6. Once the test progresses, the treadmill may go into an uphill (incline) position.
7. After a cool-down period, the patient gets off, stands still for a few seconds, and then lies down.
8. The technician administering the exam will continue to monitor the patient for blood pressure and breathing issues while

discussing any chest pain or breathing difficulty.

A stress test will last no more than fifteen minutes. The interval of the test that requires the heart to beat fast will be determined by the participant's ability to continue, and if the participant can maintain an elevated pace.

If the patient has any of the following signs or symptoms, the doctor will stop the test:

- Dizziness
- Severe panting
- High or low blood pressure
- Arrhythmia
- Chest pain
- Abnormal changes detected

The echocardiography portion of the test involves you lying down and having cold gel applied to your skin so a technician can run an ultrasound probe around your chest to get a close look at your heart and measure your valves and arteries. It's one of the easiest tests you will ever take. Lie down is the only instruction. I agreed to have these tests completed because, despite my idiocy in the past of not seeing a cardiologist with a family history of heart issues, I had learned my lesson and was determined to be more vigilant.

You believe me, right? In actuality, I had a scheduling issue one day and waited another six months before I had the tests run. Because I am young and healthy with a hint of an impatient temper, I delayed my testing yet again. Except for having a few bouts of chest discomfort in the past, and then some bad lab work, coupled with a father who died in his living room in his early sixties, there was no real rush anyway. For anyone who struggles with sarcasm in print, this is me being coy in explaining why I am a moron.

Echocardiography is a test that uses sound waves to produce live images of your heart. This image is called an echocardiogram. This test allows your physician to evaluate how your heart and valves are functioning.

What exactly did that stress test show? Nothing. You weren't expecting that, were you? It was completely normal. My resting heart rate before and after the activity showed no irregularities. No one in the room was more surprised by that than I was. I left the testing area that day relatively pleased with myself that I was not only able to stay on the treadmill for the allotted time with an elevated heart rate, but I hadn't even vomited on anyone to do it.

I'm sitting at work the day after my stress echo, not even realizing I am rubbing my left pec, when an anesthesiologist in my group asks me if my chest is hurting. It is a low-key type of nuisance, nothing so major I have given it much thought that day. The anesthesiologist casually mentions to me that he has an ultrasound probe that hooks into his phone and he could take a look at my heart. Boys love their toys.

The doctor had just gotten the probe and wanted to try it out. Can we do it? Of course, we can! The next thing I know, I am standing in an office section located near the front of the operating rooms having goop put on my chest for the second day in a row. Like a scene from a sci-fi movie, a friend of mine examines my heart with an ultrasound on his phone screen. This might sound like a futuristic episode of some sitcom you would find hard to believe, but here we were.

The anesthesiologist tells me he sees something that looks weird on his phone and asks another doctor from the group to come look at it. "Bulbous" is the term they use to describe it. The conversation in the corner parlayed into a debate to determine if it was the angle of the probe on my chest or simply the fact that we were looking at the ultrasound on a cell phone. The discussion continued for a few minutes before I was allowed to wipe the gel off my chest and put my scrub top back down. The final decision was that something looked different than normal, but it could have been an effect of the tools being used.

Whatever they think they have seen, I now believe it is time to let this anesthesiologist know I had ultrasound imaging done a day earlier, and I should probably take a look at my results to see what was found. That "bulbous" area that my brilliant coworker had found on his phone was also found on the echo portion of my testing. It turns out that I had an ascending aortic root dilation, or more simply an aneurysm that sat directly on top of my aortic valve.

Further testing would be needed for the definite sizes, but there it was. Another one of those "aha" moments. An hour ago I was the guy who took a daily pill to control my cholesterol, but passed a stress test with flying colors. Now I am suddenly the guy who has to figure out how big the aneurysm in his chest is.

Chapter 3
What Does This Even Mean?

When a physician reads a report from a radiologist that an echo or an ultrasound has shown an abnormality on an image, the next step is to order an additional imaging test that can get a closer look at anatomy. These additional tests will allow for more specific measurements of any abnormalities. Ultrasound maps the structures like a bat or a whale does by using echolocation. It isn't perfect but is a fantastic way to determine if any additional imaging needs to be done. However, depending on the angles of the probe and how it is facing certain structures, the measurement numbers can occasionally vary from the actual dimensions.

Something as simple as the positioning of the technologist's hand while freezing the image on the screen for measurement could skew the numbers up or down. This doesn't mean that the test is invalid. It only means that if a resulting number is noted that falls above certain ranges, then more specific measurements will need to be taken.

The same anesthesiologist who had seen the bulbous area in my chest with a probe on his phone mentioned this fact when we were talking about the next step. I was told the ultrasound numbers were often wrong. I felt a sense of relief for approximately thirty seconds. Then he clarified that the preliminary images from ultrasound produced measurements that were often smaller than in actuality.

I thought the good doctor was telling me not to worry because the additional testing would show the dilation to be smaller. Nope. Instead, it was some more good news. But there was no need to worry until we knew for sure that the actual size of the aneurysm was something big enough to be concerned about. There are a lot of scenarios that only require people to watch them for growth over time. Some patients watch dilations or aneurysms for a lifetime with no intervention. An individual's abnormal anatomy is not a fixed scenario where anything outside of a standard range is a surgical intervention. Not all hope was lost at the moment.

A computed tomography (CT) scan was ordered so we could get an even better idea of what we were dealing with. A cardiac computed tomography test allows for an in-depth look at internal structures. In this case, images of my heart.

A computed tomography (CT) scan combines a continuous series of X-ray images taken from different angles around your body. A computer is used to process the images to create cross-sectional images of the bones, blood vessels, and soft tissues inside your body. CT scan images provide more detailed information than plain X-rays do, allowing the user to see inside the object of the scan without cutting.

This scan allows for the specific measurements a cardiologist would use to determine if my aneurysm was the type of scenario that needed to be watched over time for growth, or if an intervention needed to be done at some point. The CT scan was scheduled for a week later after the echo results were read. There was no sense of urgency at this time because this was no big deal.

There are situations where you might find an abnormality in your heart, and you live with it without issue. I had been living with an aortic root dilation for years and didn't even know it was there. I had not felt any effects on my body. No diminished quality of life. If it hadn't been for an imaging exam, I might have never been aware of it at all.

I am not exactly a shorter man at 6'3", so there is always the chance that the size of my aorta is bigger because it corresponds to my height. Everything in life is a matter of perspective. If you have big feet, then you wear big shoes. It just makes sense. No one would ever accuse me of being a glass-half-full kind of guy, but I was trying to think positively at this point. It sounds better when I use the term positive instead of denial.

The day rolls around for my CT scan, and I show up to work, skip my morning coffee and lunch, then head over in the afternoon to have the test run. A CT machine looks like a big donut. There is a table in front of the donut that will insert you into the middle of the machine where you will lie still for the scan.

You lie on the table and get safety strapped to it like a human burrito. Your arms stay out of the security blanket burrito wrap because you will need an IV for this procedure. The CT scan can be done with or without contrast dye. For a scan of your heart, your arms will be placed above your head. Once the IV is tested, the table will slide into the donut hole where the images are taken.

For a better image with the scan, a contrast dye can be used during a CT scan. A very small percentage of patients might have a moderate reaction to contrast dye. That exact number is around the 1% mark, according to the 2012 article by Manouchehr Saljoughian, PharmD, titled

"Intravenous Radiocontrast Media: A Review of Allergic Reactions." You can find this article online in case you need some light reading for later.

Some of the symptoms of a contrast dye reaction can include vomiting or hives. My personal experience with contrast dye was not great. I vomited when the contrast dye was in, so I have started to be pretreated before receiving contrast and have not had any issues. The pretreatment is a fairly simple process with some steroids taken the night before, an additional dose the morning of the scan, and an antihistamine. If you have had sensitivity or issues in the past, you might mention that to your provider so you can have a better experience in the future.

Although you might not feel nauseous when the contrast dye is infused, prepare yourself for an extremely weird sensation when this solution is pushed into your IV. (I get a weird taste similar to salt brine in my mouth when the contrast dye is pushed.) Next, you will feel the contrast flowing through your body. It doesn't hurt, but anyone who has had it can probably describe the sensation of feeling like you have peed on yourself as it scales south while you are in full-on burrito status. The CT machine will tell you to hold your breath, but I bet you'll be more focused on holding your bladder.

The process of a computer building those images into a 3D model takes time. You will have to wait for the better part of a day before the images are constructed into a finished product and available for a radiologist to look at. Then the report has to be dictated by the radiologist, which takes more time. I just don't want you to think that when you are unstrapped from the table, someone is going to start giving you measurements from the scan. A good rule of thumb in medicine is that if something is non-emergent, then it will proceed at the roaring speed of a herd of turtles.

A CT scan is not the only test you might run into on your way to surgery. Another common procedure that you could find yourself looking forward to is a magnetic resonance imaging (MRI) scan. For thoroughness, I can walk you through what an MRI might entail based on my experience of treating people who had problems with tight spaces or holding still.

Magnetic Resonance Imaging (MRI) is an imaging technique used in radiology to form pictures of the anatomy and the physiological processes of the body using strong magnetic fields, magnetic field gradients, and radio waves to generate images of the organs in the body.

An MRI tech will ask you some questions before you head into the room with the huge door that looks as if it could withstand a fairly heavy blast. Do you have any metal in your body? Do you have issues with enclosed spaces? Have you had any eye surgery? You might not be sure if you are losing it or if the person asking the questions has lost their marbles.

The doors to MRI rooms resemble fallout shelter doors because the power of the magnets inside can be more than 30,000 times greater than what you feel daily with the gravitational pull of the Earth, according to *"The Physics of MRI Safety"* by Lawrence Panych, Ph.D., and Bruno Madore, Ph.D. Every item used in that room will have no magnetism. The staff who enter the room are asked the same questions and are patted down for keys and pens to make sure they don't create a scenario where the charting utensil in their pocket becomes a projectile. The monitors used to keep tabs on you, anesthesia machines, and even IV poles are non-magnetic. This is the reason the MRI staff will persistently ask about metal components from previous surgeries.

The donut entrance in this machine looks more like a tunnel. And depending on your size, that tunnel can get a little tight. Patients are strapped in with an IV in place, similar to the CT scan. You have to remain still for the images to be accurate, which can seem like an easy thing to do for a bit of time. However, consider that you will also need earplugs for this procedure because the machine will produce a very loud knocking noise while scanning those images.

Some patients prefer a bit of sedation to help them relax through what can be a weird experience of lying still for an extended period of time while the donut tunnel sounds like someone banging on pots and pans for the duration of the exam. While I have had MRI testing done in the past, the CT scan was all that was required of me for my measurements. If this test is required for you, assess how comfortably you can lie still while strapped to a bed in a noisy tunnel. If you are claustrophobic, this is the perfect time to grab some anxiety medication.

My results started to put my situation into perspective for me—and everyone else, for that matter. It turns out that my aneurysm measured 5.5 cm. That number probably means very little to you. It didn't even alarm me at the time. The general catch for elective surgical intervention with an aortic aneurysm is 5.0 cm, so I had some things to be addressed. The day my results were available, I had medical records print those results out and headed back to the operating room area to finish my day. At this point, I am still in the Amazon river mentality; denial.

On my way into the operative suites area of the hospital, I just happened upon a cardiac surgeon. I handed the results to him and asked what his opinion of this situation was. This is probably not how the scenario will work for you. The more anxious you get for results, the longer those hours will feel. I can only tell you to be patient because I was not, and I know how painful it was waiting to hear things.

A little background about where I work is that the hospital happens to have a phenomenal cardiac team with several surgeons whose results are top-tier. You could put their numbers up against any of the larger, more well-known facilities in the United States, and they would still ring true. No one who comes to this facility has to worry that they sacrificed quality to have their procedure close to home. The surgeons are active participants in The Society of Thoracic Surgeons' public reporting for cardiac surgical outcomes. The website is publicreporting.sts.org if you want to check surgeons in your area. I would encourage you to do so.

If you were to come to the facility where I work for a coronary artery bypass graft (CABG), transcatheter aortic valve replacement (TAVR), or any collection of cardiac surgery letters you would want to have taken care of, these cardiothoracic surgeons can do it and do it well. Here I was at work, equipped with the knowledge that these surgeons were fantastic. And I found myself handing over a radiologist synopsis of a CT scan on a person that this surgeon knew nothing about, had never been consulted on, and was not doing surgery on. For lack of a medical term, this is what's known as a dick move.

At first, the surgeon thought I was asking his opinion on whether or not I should proceed with surgery on a patient from an anesthesia perspective. I was told to be careful with pressures, and watch positioning, but everything should be fine. When I informed the surgeon that the paper in his hand had my name at the top, the realization that I was asking him something completely different set in. As busy as his day was, this surgeon was kind enough to sit down and review my images with me on the spot in the physician's lounge. He explained that I should restrict how much weight I lift and that the odds of an aortic aneurysm rupturing were very low. It was a reassuring moment.

Then this surgeon said something that caught me completely off guard. I was told that he would not (nor would anyone else in the group) perform the surgery. He would be happy to get me in touch with the people who could help and he knew some great surgeons who would take care of me. However, this was not a procedure that they did here at this facility. This statement was not as reassuring as the ones before it.

Hold up. Wait one minute. I live here. I work here. I could pick every single person involved in my care from anesthesia to the operating room nurse. Why would I want to go anywhere else? Well, it just so happened that my aortic valve was currently fine. That meant that I would need a valve-sparing procedure, also known as a David procedure. Unfortunately, that is not something that anyone in this group does. It is a procedure that is done by a considerably smaller group of surgeons.

Every cardiac procedure has a time commitment for surgeons to learn and perfect. For a procedure that focuses on a smaller class of patients, it would be unreasonable for surgeons at smaller facilities where the patient population is lower to invest time and resources into learning a specialty surgery like a David procedure. These surgeons are well-versed in replacing the valve and aorta both simultaneously because the patient population is prevalent even in smaller to mid-sized facilities. Specialty surgeries similar to this are normally found in larger facilities and teaching hospitals.

I consider myself lucky to work in health care, as well as work with a group of individuals who have a plethora of experience from many different backgrounds. Several doctors in my group have cardiac specializations in anesthesia and have trained and worked in some of the largest settings available in the nation. With coworkers who had worked at some of the most prestigious facilities in the world, I was able to circumvent the search for a surgeon.

To begin your search for a surgeon, the first thing you need to know is what type of procedure you will need. Once the surgery type is established, you need to find out who performs these surgeries in your town, the next town, or possibly the closest major metropolitan area. Once you make your list of surgeons that perform the surgery you need, head back over to the website where success rates are listed. Check into your first choice of surgeon. If you feel confident you have found the surgeon you would like, you can start the process of referrals and appointments to try and get on the surgical schedule.

My colleagues were able to assist me in finding the best surgeon for what I needed and start with the next difficult step in the process. That problem would be scheduling. Referrals can be problematic even for healthcare professionals. Learning to navigate referrals and office staff in medicine is something that can be mentally taxing because of insurance requirements, protocol, and how in-network and out-of-network channels work. Hope for a smooth process, but prepare mentally for an arduous journey of phone calls and long holds.

Within a day of asking for help, a coworker had contacted a friend many states away, who in turn spoke to a surgeon who agreed to look over my images. I do not say this to brag about how easily things went for me. This is more of a warning that when it comes to getting your place in line, prepare yourself for many frustrating calls. Keep a notepad handy and take meticulous notes. Write down the name of the person you spoke with, the time of the call, and what was talked about, as well as any additional numbers of people you were referred to. This will help you stay organized and retain your sanity.

My next task was to get copies of every test or image that I had completed sent to a new surgeon's office in another state. A collection of information was needed that would give him a picture of what was going on with my health and how he might be able to help me. This was an easy enough step accomplished by heading back to medical records at the hospital.

Medical records are a group of people at a hospital or clinic who can access any information in the system on a patient if a procedure was done at the facility. If you have proper identification, they can get copies of physician reports, make CD copies of images, and print anything you would need to send to someone else at a different facility. All of this can happen very quickly if you stop by with the proper ID and ask nicely. Then you can move on to the next step of sending it all away.

I sent an envelope of test results and scans to the office of the surgeon I didn't know who was several states away. The package was sent to an address given to me on a picture of a business card, that was texted to someone else, who then forwarded it to me. This is how things normally work, right? All I had to do was wait. Easy stuff. Don't lift anything too heavy, avoid vagaling (which is basically what happens when you bear down in the bathroom), and keep working until the doctor called to tell me how long I would have until I needed to do something about this dilation. Dilation sounds much more innocent than an aneurysm, don't you think?

I didn't hear anything the first week. I called the surgeon's office to confirm that the package had been received. The envelope was there but had not been looked at just yet. The second week of waiting, the surgeon went on vacation. That little detail meant that nothing was going to happen until he got back. In the third week, the surgeon was in the office and able to look at the results. And a few days into that week, he did that exact thing. He looked at the results.

I was working in surgery, talking to an orthopedic surgeon and his crew about waiting for results when my phone buzzed. Someone had left a voicemail. I had not been concerned about the time waiting because, at this point, I was still assuming that I would be watching for the growth of my aorta over time. This surgeon could tell me how long I could wait until my next scan to monitor things. It might be six months, then stretch out to a year if things stayed consistent.

That voicemail would turn out to be the cardiac surgeon's secretary saying he would like to schedule a time to chat with me. I called her back after my case had ended and asked about a time that would be convenient for him. I was informed he was currently available and within a minute, the surgeon I had never met was on the line. How nice that he was waiting for my call back.

The surgeon was discussing the measurements of the aneurysm and how these calculations are taken, talking very calmly about what would need to happen in the future. The future. A time so far off this term is used because no one wants to constrain it with a date. So I casually asked, "How long do you think it will be before I have to worry about surgery?" The pause on the line was the same that has probably been heard a million times by those who ask stupid questions because they are ignorant or unwilling to accept the truth. The answer, "Immediately." The surgeon wasn't calling to discuss future scans. This call was the surgery call. I guess that's why the surgeon made it.

The rest of the conversation was a blur. A scheduling person was going to call me back later. My work pager was going off, summoning me for the next case. I was thanking him for his time as he had just shown me some real estate while I asked a coworker to cover my room for me. It is this moment in the scenario where you need to be certain you have an excellent support system in place. You can't plan for a call like this. You could be grocery shopping or picking up your kids from school. Everything else stops at that moment.

I was at the hospital administering anesthesia like any other day. Who do you go to when you are at work? I had told maybe five people in my group what had been going on with me throughout this entire process. I walked to the office of one of those people. This physician was talking with another doctor in the group who had no idea anything was going on with my health. I sat on the couch in his office and told him I was going to have open-heart surgery. Then I started to cry.

I don't know how most grown men at your job would respond if another grown man came in and started crying all over them. The poor anesthesiologist who knew nothing about it asked if he should leave. I assured the doctor that it was fine if he stayed, and he quickly caught up with the current situation with my heart. The fact that I cried in front of two grown men doesn't make me soft or weak. It's when I get teary-eyed from sappy movies that define me that way.

Open-heart surgery is a scary thing. If you don't think so, then you have no idea what is going to happen to you. Maybe that is why you got this book. Perhaps you want to have a better idea and a healthy respect for what is going to transpire throughout this experience. But my response, the response of a man who spends every workday in surgery putting people to sleep, was to cry.

My mind raced about what this would mean for work and staffing, what it would mean financially for my family, and how my family would be forced into a scenario where the outcome isn't guaranteed. It was a lot to deal with at that moment, and I cried at work to a coworker who was probably thinking he didn't sign up for any of this. There was nothing in his job description that details babysitting emotional coworkers.

Despite the lack of job requirements to do so, these two anesthesiologists calmed me down, assured me that everything would be fine, and sent me home to talk to my wife and kids about what was happening. A single phone call changed my entire perspective. The rest of my life started at that moment. All I had to do was plan out the next six months of my existence in very specific detail. I had to make preparations I had never considered until now. And before any of that happened, I had to tell my wife the news.

Chapter 4
Make Some Plans

This is the part of the story where the rubber meets the road for preparation. I don't mean the part where you have to tell your wife that immediate surgery is in your future or you could die suddenly like your father. Instead, this is the actual planning that is involved in getting ready for that surgery. For me, there was plenty of time to get things in order. My phenomenal surgeon has a schedule that confirms his awesomeness. When scheduling called me, I received the next available surgical slot, which happened to be three months down the road. That is plenty of time to dot all the T's and cross all the I's. If you think that's backward, you obviously haven't dealt with insurance and health care. Trust me, there will be very little that is straightforward when planning for this surgery.

The majority of people who are having to make plans for major heart surgery don't fall into the same age group that I happened to be in at the time. It does happen, but it isn't the norm. That being said, there are still a lot of plans that need to be arranged for a surgery of this size. A quick checklist of things to do for surgery preparation is below.

- Talk to your employer about time off.
- Talk to your insurance provider about pre-approval requirements.
- Do you have a short-term disability policy? Talk to that provider.
- Do you have pets? Make arrangements for them.
- Stop your mail or have it picked up.
- Is there a homeowners association that will be angry if your grass isn't cut?
- Arrange for bills to be paid in advance or drafted while you are away.
- Make travel arrangements for a hotel if you aren't local.
- Any family that will be assisting you, this list will apply to them as well.
- Pack clothing for postoperative success.
- Make a worst-case scenario plan.

This doesn't seem like a small list! Some of the things on this list might seem silly. I know you were going to take care of all these things without me telling you about it. Perhaps some of the items listed above are not as simple as they would appear at first glance. We will cover some of them in a bit more detail to highlight the thought process that needs to go into major surgery preparations.

You want to talk to your employer about time off if you are still working. How much time off? How rigorous is your job? What are the lifting or weight requirements? A lot of people are surprised by how much they actually do on a daily basis when it comes to lifting. When you are done with your surgery, there is a period of time when you need your sternum to heal.

With that initial period of healing comes a weight restriction on things that can be lifted. The surgery can also come with some range-of-motion restrictions. When you are told that you need to not lift more than ten pounds for the next six weeks, how will you handle it? A gallon of milk weighs eight pounds for comparison. There is more to a successful recovery than waking up postoperatively. As time goes by, the weight restrictions will increase. Does your job require you to lift more than twenty pounds?

You now know that stocking shelves is out because you won't be allowed to lift your arms above your head. You can only lift ten pounds, so moving furniture or hay bales is done for a bit too. How long do you need to ask for to recover? How much time do you have to take off? Paid time off is great, but few people have months of stored-up paid time off. If you happen to have that much time, great! You will definitely need plenty of time.

It will take approximately three months for your sternum to fully heal. At some point on a follow-up visit, your weight restriction will climb to twenty pounds, then possibly fifty pounds. This is an individual healing process, so there will be no hard and fast time limit to plan for. Just because a restriction has been lifted, it does not mean that you suddenly have the strength or endurance to resume full activities at work. Does your job have a part-time role for you? What about light-duty positions? If the answer is no, then you and your employer need to discuss what exactly you will be able to do and when. Additionally, you will need to determine how you will manage the financial aspect of being off work for an extended amount of time.

Your employer now knows that you need surgery. Does your insurance carrier? You probably won't be the one to tell them, but you will need to follow up and make sure that everything is approved promptly before tests are done and bills start rolling in. An example of why it is important to stay on top of things came to light before I was needing to worry about surgery. During the testing phase, the cardiologist said that due to my family history and age, I needed a stress test with an echo. My insurance company decided that his opinion was a little too progressive for them, so they approved the stress test, but no imaging.

If you recall, it was the imaging that saved my life. Without the image that shows an aortic root aneurysm sitting directly above my aortic valve, I move on with my daily activities believing there are no issues with my heart. I assume that since all my results were normal from the stress test, I have nothing to worry about. I don't worry for one second because I am young(ish) and relatively delusional about my health.

My life moves forward the same as it always has right up until the moment the aneurysm dissects and kills me. That might sound a bit dramatic, but this will be the first lesson in self-advocacy that I can teach you. No one in your life wants to see you healthier more than you. With that being said, you now know who will need to put in the work on the treadmill after surgery, and on the phone with insurance carriers who deny testing your physician has requested. A test might seem redundant or confusing to you, but that doesn't mean it isn't necessary. I can assure you that there aren't any cardiologists making their living off of echocardiogram profits.

I won't go into the ridiculous nature of insurance providers overruling medical professionals and dictating care. I will tell you to be vigilant and make sure your insurance carrier will be covering all the tests and procedures you need to be done so you aren't left holding the bill for portions of the process when surgery is all over. Your insurance provider will probably act surprised and tell you that some of the tests that were requested might be unnecessary. Rest assured that your insurance provider has seen these tests and covered them many times before.

Do you believe the line that a second opinion from a different physician is required to approve the testing that was submitted? Of course not. But occasionally an inconvenience to the patient can monopolize time and patience and save the insurer the cost of the test because people will give up. Do not give up. When you get angry at the process, remember that a huge process is exactly what it is. You should envision yourself as the star of a grand production, where everything that happens is focused on making sure you get all the attention you deserve. While individuals love to believe they are the headliner of a huge show, it is normally a surprise for people when they find out the show is actually a circus.

Another insurance company you might need to talk to is the one providing your short-term disability if you have it. This is a plan that you can purchase or may have been purchased by your employer, that covers a portion of your pay when you are out of work for a certain amount of time. Plans vary, so you will need to check on the specifics of what you have and can expect from your provider and a time frame to expect it. The paperwork will normally involve three sections: one for you, one for your surgeon, and one for your employer. The insurance company will need all three returned to them before processing the claim. Even if you believe you are doing the right thing, it can sometimes come back and bite you. This is yet another lesson I learned the hard way.

My portion of the short-term disability paperwork asked me when I thought I might be able to return to work. I am an optimistic guy, and it asked when I thought, so I put a date two months after my surgery date with a question mark. That date turned out to be wrong. Very, very wrong. How was I supposed to know? This was my first heart surgery as a patient. In anesthesia, our time with the patient ends in the operating room, and everyone leaves to have a great life immediately after we walk away. At least that is what we all like to believe. Anesthesia doesn't continuously follow our patients through the postoperative phase for weeks (or months) into the recovery phase.

Sure enough, eight weeks after my surgery, the checks stopped coming. The short-term disability company had not called me, had not called the surgeon to see if I was cleared, and had not even called my employer to see if I was back to work. They just stopped the checks. When I called to ask about the lack of payments, I was told that I was the one who put the date back to work on the paperwork. This was true. There was no denying it. The question mark didn't matter. When I asked why they hadn't checked with anyone to see if I had been cleared to return to work, I was told the company didn't have the personnel to check on all claims. I always assumed that was part of the job of the claim handler, but I learned that wasn't true. Thanks to that little fact, I got to fill out the paperwork again to get it all re-approved.

Eventually, it was re-approved. It only took the company seven weeks to reapprove my claim. That was seven weeks the disability company didn't pay me while they determined if my not being at work from the same surgery that was approved the first time was legitimate. Eventually, the payments were reinstated. A week after they were reinstated, payments were stopped a second time. This time the reason was because of a lack of a follow-up appointment date. Weeks went by without answers and without payments again.

My adjuster was called the third time payment was stopped, and she said she needed to speak to a nurse to verify that the progress note from a cardiac surgeon was accurate. You heard that right. The insurance company is going to verify with a nurse that they employ if the progress note from a cardiothoracic surgeon met the disability carrier's standard for continued payment. After a week of waiting, my wife called back to find out she hadn't bothered to call the nurse yet. After a few ill-advised but apparently very effective phrases from my wife, the adjuster had it approved that same day.

Remember this story when you assume that anyone involved in making payments to you (or for you) when the time comes for surgery actually cares if it happens promptly. Or if the payments happen at all, for that matter. Leave the section blank that asks when you will be back to work because honestly, you have no idea. A good rule of thumb is that no matter what any insurance provider tells you, or how friendly your claims handler sounds on the phone, these companies are in business to make money.

That is the whole point of collecting your premiums. Actuaries have calculated certain risks for the market, and every dollar they pay out cuts into profitability. You should never assume that someone who is spending money on you wants to do it. If given the opportunity, the person writing the checks will stop making payments as soon as possible. It isn't fair. It definitely isn't fun. However, these are the hoops that you will be required to jump through. Are you starting to get excited yet?

Once the paperwork is done, it's time to manage the household. Arrange for pets, bills, and housework to be taken care of before you leave town. Your house could be empty for a few weeks, but life will carry on even while you are lying in the hospital. Also, let the people who are assisting you know that once you are back home, there is a possibility you could still need some help with these things. Just because you have managed to get back to town does not mean you will be pushing a lawnmower around anytime soon. If you have large pets like I do, one accidental jump on your chest from a big dog can send you back to the hospital.

There has never been a better time in your life to tap into your network of friends and family. Have you ever heard the saying, "Many hands make light work"? Don't be afraid to ask people for small things and big things. Don't be afraid to let them know you don't want it, but rather you need it. There are no awards at the end of this for doing as much of it alone as possible. Mistakes can lead to increased recovery times. No one wants that. If you are the type of person who has a hard time asking for help, this is a great time for a little personal growth. Grow right towards asking for help. You will want it, and you will definitely need it.

Have you ever been late on a payment before? Sometimes a bill can get dropped between the seat and the console in your car. Suddenly, you get a call from the company wondering where their money is. While this is completely an accident, you still get embarrassed. Now imagine that happening with your house payment, car payment, and electric bill all at the same time. For a person like me, that is nightmare fuel. Not the kind of activity you want to be dealing with postoperatively.

Let me ask you what type of relationship you have with your bank. Do you think they are very concerned about your heart surgery? Ask your banker and find out. I bet your banker will say, "Oh no" and "I hope everything goes well." They will probably tell you about someone they know who had a procedure as well. Hugs might be in order.

Then, if you are brave or have a weird sense of humor, ask them how long they will be delaying payments without reporting them to the credit bureaus. Watch the expression of concern turn to confusion, and then the babbling excuses start to flow. The answer is zero. Arrange for your bills in advance. Make sure your spouse or whoever is helping you knows what is due and when. You can set up an autopay system. If you have the means, you could even pay it in advance. Do whatever is necessary to be confident you won't receive any stressful calls during your recovery period.

Along with bills, stopping your mail or having a trusted person pick it up is just a good way to avoid letting strangers know you are gone from your house for an extended period. I didn't think a house robbery would help with the stress levels of recovery, so I decided to try and avoid it. I don't want to tell you how to live your life, but cataloging stolen household items for the police seemed like more than what I was wanting to deal with the minute I came home from the hospital.

If you are in town, maybe this isn't a concern for you. What happens if you travel a state away and some hiccup keeps you there for a couple of weeks? It is easier to be safe and have someone check the mail and water the plants than to come home to shattered glass or a broken door jam. It sounds like I live in a pretty shady neighborhood. I don't, but I just like to plan for worst-case possibilities. If you stress the little things before the surgery, you can relax about most things after the surgery.

Once you have a surgical date and the insurance has agreed to pay for it, a lot of people will need to make some arrangements for a place to stay for the surgery. There is always the chance your procedure will take place at your local hospital. If that is the case, be happy and skip right over this step. Lucky for you. However, for the people who do have to travel, even if it is only a town over, you will need to make some plans for a hotel.

As soon as you know your surgical date, call ahead and find out availability. You never know if there will be a softball tournament in town, a business meeting, or even a miniature railroad conductors' convention. Maybe the city you are going to is a vacation hotspot. I went to Cleveland, which I never considered a must-see destination. Yet, there were very few hotels in the city with availability the week of spring break when I had my surgery. Hotels can fill up fast, so grab a spot as soon as you know your date.

When booking lodging, location can be important. Consider trying to make things easy for the family to come and go because there will be a lot of coming and going to the hospital normally. Visitation times in the ICU are sporadic, and surgery schedules can run long. I decided to grab a place that was connected to the heart hospital by an enclosed, elevated walkway. I did this so it would be convenient for my wife to get back and forth to see me after surgery. The joke was on me because when I arrived for testing the day before my surgery in late March 2020, the hospital shut down the walkways and entrances for Covid-19.

That's right. I had my open-heart procedure at the beginning of the pandemic. My wife and three kids are in a hotel room they can't leave and a walkway they can't use for an extended couple of weeks. It seems like a surefire recipe for disaster. Some people are just born lucky. I will touch more on that later. The spoiler alert is that we came home with everyone we left with, and no one was beaten or eaten in the hotel room. With three kids ages sixteen, fourteen, and seven, we chalk that up as a win.

Another thing you might not be thinking about is your wardrobe. This is not a reference to what type of slacks you wear to meet the surgeon the day before you get cracked. This is a postoperative scenario you have not thought of before. Once you get your zipper installed, you can't just start pulling shirts over your head. Those arms will be staying low for a bit, so you need to look into some button-up pajama tops. And when you go to buy these button-up tops, buy them big. You won't need anything form-fitting or tight to apply pressure to the incision site on your chest. Buy a bathrobe to throw on if you get chilly. Try to find some house shoes that you can slip on your feet that have some grip on the bottom. You want to minimize bending over to put on shoes, and you want something on your feet that will keep your floor from turning into an ice-skating rink.

Think of ways to stay safe and comfortable for weeks after you get home. Remove tripping hazards around the house like large rugs that could catch your foot. You might rearrange furniture if there is a coffee table that always bangs your shin when you walk by. Clear and open pathways are considerably more important than the feng shui of the Ficus plant to the doorway. Safety is key when you have a healing incision that can't support trauma. Imagine yourself as a toddler learning to walk for the first time. Plan for short trips that involve straight lines and a lack of things that could knock you off balance.

These are all things for you to consider when the time starts to roll around for your surgical day. This list is probably far from inclusive of everything, but it will help you get the ball rolling for preparation and not be caught off guard. You know what they say about the best-laid plans, right? Expect a few hiccups and be prepared to roll with it. When you think you are ready for everything, that is when you might get thrown for a loop like I did. Prepare as best you can, and then deal with whatever comes up.

Once you have planned for payments and pets, hotels, and house shoes, it's time to plan for something a little different. What is a worst-case-scenario plan? I know no one wants to talk about this, but I think it might be the most important thing anyone can do for themselves or their family. What happens if things go bad? Does everyone in your household know what to do or what your wishes are? This is much bigger than a will or a trust. That is simply asset allocation. This is the section where I will explain what I did to prepare my wife for the worst scenario imaginable. While uncomfortable, to avoid this situation could create a stressful predicament when it's too late for the people you love the most.

To help me organize my thoughts, I prepared a living document. I am using the term living document to explain that I wrote a continuously revisable list of everything I could think of at the time. Then I left the document stored where I could go back to it repeatedly as I remembered additional things to add to it. In this document, I put some step-by-step instructions for what my wife would need to do if I was in the highly unlikely situation of not making it off the table or out of the hospital. I wanted it easy to find and hard to lose, so I created an online document where it could be saved and updated regularly from anywhere I had internet access. All my wife had to do was sit at my computer, log in, and look at the documents under my profile. My wife knew my login, but I put it on a sticky note anyway. You know, stress and all.

My wife and I had talked about the fact that I was preparing this document, but she only wanted to know of its existence, not so much its contents. This is the same woman who wanted to know I was having surgery, but not too much about it. She did ask me how she would know which document was the one she should read when she logged on since there were multiple things there. I made it as easy as possible. I titled the document "What to do when I'm dead." She was not amused. Understandable, but I wasn't kidding. Make it easy. If this situation arises, do you think anyone is in the state of mind to be looking around for something you have named cleverly? "The Rise and Fall of the Household Emperor" might seem funny to you at the time but might not catch the attention of a loved one dealing with a very stressful scenario.

What exactly needs to be in this document? Well, that depends on some very personal details of your current situation. I was younger than a lot of people having open heart surgery, so I have three kids still in the house. (One of my children is a bit younger than the first two. We refer to him affectionately by his nickname, "Oops.") While my wife might be well aware of the location of the bank accounts that she pays bills from, she has no idea where investment accounts are located and who she should contact. When your spouse calls, would they know what to ask about investments and 401k accounts and what would have to be done with them? If not, walk your spouse through it on the document. A clear step-by-step process will be appreciated by anyone who has little knowledge of investment accounts and the like.

With my children, social security documents would have to be filed. No one has ever dealt with that in my household. Perhaps you need to look into some processes and how to accomplish some things yourself and then outline them for the people who need to know them. I know that I did. The beautiful thing about online documents is that you can hyperlink, which means you can copy and paste a web address right into the document. That makes it simple to just click on it and go where you need to be as you are working through the outline. I put a web address in the document with the statement "You need to call these people about life insurance", and then bam— names, addresses, and phone numbers are all embedded there. This makes it simple for my wife to get these things done.

Imagine teaching a child to tie their shoes. You don't say, tie your shoes. If you do, read this section twice. You need to explain in detail every step in the process to get things done if you are not around to help. Don't gloss over steps. Don't say you have life insurance unless you are telling them where, what type, who to call, their phone number, and what to do when receiving the benefit. If you believe they might have questions, link a tax guy you trust to answer those questions. If you don't know something and have to look it up, don't just put the answer in the document. Write the steps you took and where you went to find the answer.

What are some additional things you might need in this document? I am not a wealth planner or an attorney, so I will tell you some of the major items I put in my document. This is going to be personally tailored to your life. Life insurance is a great jumping-off point. Include all the information mentioned earlier, with additional information linking them to how to get death certificates that will be required in filing for any of those life insurance plans, and everything else for that matter. Do you have investment and retirement accounts? Where are they, and who does your family need to call? Will they have to change owner information or remove certain money and move it elsewhere? Who do you want to help them with any questions they have? What is the best course of action to make sure the money lasts? If you haven't already, it might be a good time to meet with an advisor to help you structure a way to ensure your family's financial health.

Do you own boats and toys that no one else drives or knows how to park? Should they be sold? How do you renew the tags if they will be kept? Who do you go to for maintenance? What do you want to be done with your body? Are you a cremation or burial kind of person? Do you have a plot? Do you care about one? What organization will handle the arrangements? What is the average amount for a funeral these days? Are you donating your whole body to science to save on the cost of a funeral? These are all the types of things that need to be placed in an easy-to-find document with answers and links. If you are lucky like me, you have a spouse that is very astute when it comes to technical stuff. I deposit money in the bank, and things just happen for me at the house. The lights come on, there is food in the pantry, and there are current tags on vehicles. I consider myself a lucky guy, except for the whole aneurysm thing.

If you do have kids, make sure your spouse knows the proper agencies to contact about social security and the benefits afforded to your children and for how long. Make sure your spouse knows how to file paperwork to collect your benefits.

Later in life, there is the possibility to switch social security plans if the amount that has been growing untouched will be a greater amount than the spousal amount. There are lots of informative sections on the government website. It is an easy web address to remember as well. It is simply ssa.gov. You might want to stop by to get yourself acclimated to what is possible for everyone in your family. I know that I did.

Spend some time reflecting on what you take care of in the household, and that the person you would be leaving behind will be responsible for all of those things. This includes everything from vehicle licensing to property taxes. This can take some time, but it doesn't need to be done all at once. Things can pop into your head, and having something online makes it that much easier to amend it. As long as your spouse is okay with it, have an open line of communication about the activities that need to happen. If you have older children, this is a great time to walk them through the situations they will be facing as adults. Can they check their oil, change a tire, or open a bank account? This is a great way to get the focus off of the surgery and spend quality time with your family.

On a personal note, while you are planning for a future that you aren't a part of, make sure you are participating in the time leading up to the trip. Don't be the person who plans for the worst-case scenario so much that you miss out on some great moments with your family before you have surgery. This ordeal will leave you sore and unable to do a lot of those things when you get back home. It is your responsibility to plan for the worst, but this is your opportunity to bring joy and love in the moments leading up to surgery. It is a stressful time. Just be mindful of that and try not to let it dictate your days with your family. Be loving and kind. Remember, these are the people writing your eulogy.

Now that we've covered the morbid planning, we can get back to the positive side of things and what needs to be done to move toward recovery. Things go well far more often than not, so preparation is not a concession to an untimely end. If anyone realizes that the time they have been spending with their family needs to be increased, then all of the planning is a success whether a document is created or not. Do not be discouraged or sad when you make plans that seem scarily finite. You buy life insurance because at some point you will die. You don't spend your days mulling over your demise. You just made a plan and kept living. The same principle applies before surgery. Robert Breault said, "Enjoy the little things in life, for one day you may look back and realize they were the big things."

Chapter 5
Let's Take a Trip

As I mentioned earlier, my surgery was not scheduled at the facility where I work. There was going to be some travel involved, as I was having my procedure done in Cleveland, Ohio. I don't live in Cleveland. I don't even live in Ohio. The plan was that I was going to fly down to Cleveland alone, and then my wife was going to meet me a couple of days later when she arrived with our children. There was school to attend for the kids, and dogs to drop off at boarding, and I was just scheduled to have some testing done in the days leading up to surgery. This was no problem. We had it all planned out. My wife wasn't a huge fan of me being alone, but I assured her that I was a big boy and could manage a flight and taxi ride on my own. I had done it before, so I was confident I could pull it off before my surgery as well.

If you haven't already guessed, none of that happened. As the date got closer, the numbers for Covid-19 got larger. People were starting to take notice, and before you knew it, the schools in our area were closed. My kids were now home with online learning and nowhere to go with all after-school activities canceled. I had a plane ticket, but did I want to risk an infection unnecessarily right before this major surgery? A friend of mine was worried about my exposure and was prepared to drive me down to Cleveland so I wouldn't be in airports. The situation with a new virus was all brand new. This means that my family had some decisions to make.

Perhaps there is a group of people reading this right now who are probably red-in-the-face angry because I didn't want to get on a plane because of Covid-19. Maybe the numbers were inflated, maybe it was a hoax, or maybe history will show something else. This story isn't about the political landscape of American politics in 2020. This is about having open heart surgery in the initial days of a pandemic when nothing was known for certain. When you are going to have open heart surgery, you are required to go to the dentist and get clearance to make sure no mouth bacteria are going to sneak up on you unknowingly. Do not get distracted by the fact that I am talking about changing plans because of a disease that was unknown at the time and had no defined course of treatment. We are all just going to move on.

Pushing forward is what we did as a household. A family meeting determined that since the kids were out of school and my job said that I can't afford to get sick this close to surgery and sent me home, we were all driving to

Cleveland together. The plan changed and was moved forward overnight. You can't linger on the changes that have to be made. You can only roll with it and pack a bag. We dropped off some furry friends at our boarding place of choice, loaded the car, and set out together on a trip to Cleveland.

My wife and I had tossed around saving a little money on hotels by reserving one across campus from the heart hospital. This would require her to walk back and forth from the hotel to the hospital. The hospital campus is quite large, so I didn't want her to navigate the streets when she might be stressed. Instead, I opted for a more expensive choice that was connected to the heart hospital by a sky bridge walkway. I wanted her to feel comfortable coming and going during my stay so she could relax if possible and not feel like she was too far away. Are you sensing how considerate I am at this point? The fear of surgery had nothing to do with it, I am sure.

We called ahead to the hotel and confirmed that our room would have a small refrigerator and a microwave. These items would allow us to bring food for preparation in the hotel. Feeding a growing teenage boy is similar to owning a Bengal tiger, so we wanted options. These room items were confirmed, so we loaded a van full of food and clothes to make our way to the beautiful city of Cleveland, Ohio, from Wisconsin. This is just a quick little ten-hour drive with the family.

When you have a long trip and something is clouding the air, try to be open in communication with the people you are with and answer questions honestly. If you are scared, chances are that they are too. My family was very open about the procedure at hand. Some family members liked looking at the pictures of the actual surgery online, while others preferred to keep their food on the inside. Try to remember that there are very few wrong ways to handle a stressful environment. Some methods might be more productive than others, but the best approach should involve being accepting of how people choose to cope with that scenario.

If someone wants to deal with stress in silence, do not feel like you need to push them to open up before they are ready. That silence could be the only thing keeping that person from an explosion of emotion. If you have someone who suddenly feels inclined to plan out every detail of the next six months, go ahead and let them. The focus of coping with stress is accepting whatever the coping mechanism is and trying to find a positive element that you can work with. Then you can work together to help an individual grow and feel accepted. Let people know you are available to them. Then be available.

When we arrived at the hotel in Cleveland, a couple of things immediately caught our attention once in the room. There was no microwave for cooking food. The refrigerator was technically there, but it was filled to 90% capacity with mini-bar essentials. We rolled with it. Five people, two weeks' worth of snacks and clothes, and all the electronics needed to complete school work on the road were all tucked into a single room with two queen beds. To be honest, I was kind of glad I wasn't staying in that room the whole time in Cleveland. Despite a few hiccups, we were still in Cleveland. The next day would begin the actual surgical journey.

Would it be a benefit to get mad and yell and scream because the hotel told us something that wasn't true? Would that help the stress level of my children? Of course not. This was just another hoop we would jump through if it meant we were still moving toward our goal. Always try to focus on the end result. You shouldn't drive a car watching just in front of the hood. Keep your eyes down the road to avoid being reactionary at every small bump. Your family is in this for the long haul, so try and keep the focus a little farther down the road. My family settled into the room, and we tried to take our minds off the reason we were there.

The first day at the heart hospital is packed with blood work and testing. New images are taken to monitor any changes that might be occurring. In my case, I met with several people whom a lot of patients might not meet. Because my father had passed away from a heart event, and I was diagnosed at a younger age, I was meeting with a geneticist. This doctor would walk me through all of the things that my blood work would and could show in the way of inheritable traits for heart issues such as these. This is not something that most people will need to worry about if there is not a clear historical reason for genetic testing.

If you are the first person in your family to have a heart condition, then the likelihood of having a genetic trait that could be passed on to your children could be as high as 30 percent. This statistic is according to a collaborative study involving the Icahn School of Medicine at Mount Sinai, the German Heart Center Munich, AstraZeneca, and Karolinska Institutet in Sweden. Different inheritable conditions run at different rates of manifestation. Coronary artery disease, one of the largest global killers, is inherited by less than a quarter of those who have the condition. While high cholesterol has higher inheritability rates, this condition is significantly easier to control if caught early.

Why wouldn't physicians test everyone? This is a complicated question that has further-reaching implications than those we are covering here for heart surgery. One of the main reasons is money. Someone has to pay for this testing, which can be expensive. Some insurance companies are more willing to ante up for genetic testing when there's a clear historical precedent. If it is important for you to know the heritability of your condition for the security of your family members, you need to contact a geneticist and speak with them about the specifics of having blood work done to look at the twenty-plus genes currently being monitored for heart disease.

This is a blessing and a curse in my personal opinion. I know exactly what I have to deal with and what needs to happen to correct it. This test can find markers that will tell me if my sibling or my children need to be monitored for the same type of issue based on a trait that I could have passed on. I spent three months waiting on my appointment for this surgery with the thought of passing this issue to my children hanging over my head. It affected my sleep, my stress levels, and every other facet of my existence at that time. While speaking with the geneticist, I became very scared for my children.

What if I had unknowingly passed a trait on to one of my kids? For the rest of their lives, each of them would have to be tested for anomalies and monitored if they tested positive. The problem would be hanging over their heads, not for three months, but instead their entire lives. It suddenly dawned on me what some children and families are forced to deal with when children learn at an early age that they have a debilitating condition. The fear for my children was more debilitating than any concern I had for my own surgery.

If my children have inherited a cardiac issue from me, there would be treatment plans and lifelong follow-ups. My children would be forced to come to grips with things well beyond their years and beyond their control. The thought of what my children's lives could become scared me. As a parent, one of the main focuses of my life has been trying to provide an easier route for my children than the one I had growing up. I think this is a common notion among parents.

My blood was drawn that would be sent to the lab for testing. The meeting with the geneticist was on the first day, but those results wouldn't be back for several weeks. Just a tiny little extra something to occupy a section of your mind while you are preparing to have your chest sawed open. The meeting with the geneticist was informative. This doctor will be trying to build a family tree of health history, so before you have this appointment, it might be a good idea to try and find out what the people in your family died from and at what age. This is the basis for determining risk factors and approximating applicable statistics.

I was not as prepared as I should have been but still did relatively well on my family's history of diseases and causes of death. If you don't happen to know what your maternal grandmother died from and when it happened, make some calls before you show up for this meeting. Fortunately, every single marker came back negative for me. I felt a sense of relief believing I was just unlucky and my kids weren't necessarily forced into a lifetime of treatment plans and testing. All my kids would still be required to have baseline echos, but this was still good news at the time. The caveat I will add here is that even though all my markers came back negative, one of my kids did still have an anomaly on the echo. The details are for my family, but the takeaway here is that genetic testing is a probabilities game. There are no certainties.

The first full day in Cleveland was a busy one. Bouncing from one desk to the next all day long and weaving my way in and out of crowds of people doing the same thing. This heart hospital is a monstrosity. Floors of check-ins and different areas, servicing thousands of people every day. This hospital is also a well-oiled machine. I managed to stay on the schedule they had sent me weeks earlier in my surgery packet. I was never behind for check-in times at the following appointment despite the throngs of people needing to be seen in each area.

If you have spent any time in a hospital in your entire life, you understand what an accomplishment staying on schedule is. As my day ended, I started my journey back to the hotel room to share my concerns with my family. We like to talk through everything as a group. No one needs to feel left out because everyone's opinion is important. My mind was racing with all the activity that happened on day one.

I made my way into the walkway that connects the heart hospital to my hotel, where I was met by a hodgepodge of medical practitioners at one level or another. Everyone at the table had masks and hand sanitizer. They were pack hunters, surrounding anyone who approached the walkway and asked if they were an employee or guest, dispensing alcohol onto hands, and explaining to rub together vigorously. The walkways were now being monitored, and only employees or patients were allowed to use them. The entrance to my hotel had been closed, so that was no longer an option for coming and going to the hospital. Yet again, all of my planning had been met with failure. My wife was going to have to walk around the block to get into the hospital to see me, or so I thought.

The hospital in Cleveland was fast to respond to Covid-19 and shut down the majority of entrances. By the afternoon of my first day, entry to the hospital was restricted to patients and providers. Even those who were allowed in could only enter through a fraction of the normal routes of entry. Security had been positioned at all points in and out, and signs had already been printed and placed directing traffic and informing people that their families were no longer allowed in the building. You heard that correctly. I was now having open heart surgery in a strange city with an unfamiliar hospital during a pandemic, and my wife and kids were not allowed in the hospital to see me before or after.

The caution tape at the designated entrance steered you toward people with masks, hand sanitizer, and thermometers. A staff member pointed you to the alcohol station while another came at you with a temperature probe. All of this happened simultaneously while bombarding you with questions of where you have been, who you have been in contact with, and how you are feeling. Again, things had completely changed in the blink of an eye.

My second day of tests and appointments was the polar opposite of my first day. All the employees were still there, manning their desks in their designated areas. All the chairs were there too, filling expansive waiting areas where patients would pause, listening for their name to be called, and moving on to the next step of the itinerary that was mailed out to them. But those chairs were empty today. Staff asked my name and birthday, what I was there for, and then ushered me right in. There was a line of people at the entrance that I can only assume were employees, because everywhere I went in the hospital once inside was a ghost town. I saw less than ten other patients the entire day. I was three hours ahead of schedule by the end of the day because, in most areas, I was the only person currently on the schedule.

While I was running around getting tested the day before, oblivious to what was happening behind the scenes, the hospital had closed off access and canceled all elective testing and procedures. It was like a post-apocalyptic movie without the zombies. Empty rooms and patient-less areas everywhere I went. People waved to me and called my name because I was the only name on the list for the entire morning schedule.

It was a bit eerie, to say the least. However, today was a big day for me. Since the initial portion of my scheduling was all done by phone, I was meeting my surgeon for the first time before he was set to operate on me the next day. That shouldn't be the way it goes for most people. You will meet the doctor in advance. Yet, nothing about my surgery was going very normal at this point.

A schedule for a patient showing up for heart surgery might look something like what is listed below...

Day 1
Cardiology Registration
Radiology - Chest X-ray
Electrocardiogram
Routine Labs and Bloodwork
Genetic Healthcare
Cardiologist Review
Pulmonary Function Lab
Echocardiogram

Day 2
Thoracic Clinic
Cardiothoracic Preoperative Clearance
Anesthesia Clearance
Meet your Cardiac Surgeon

Day 3
Surgery Day

My surgeon is a very personable fellow, whose likability is only overshadowed by his talent. Because of his talent, his schedule tends to be a bit of a waiting contest if you aren't the type of patient that needs to be seen immediately due to your condition. When he agreed that my surgery was a priority, I still waited over three months to get my day on the schedule. You could fall into one of several categories for surgery. There are emergent, urgent, and elective categories to determine the speed that a patient needs to be scheduled. In this case, these classifications are determined by the condition of your heart and overall health.

Some people were worried about the wait being three months. Occasionally, the person was me, but time did help when it came to planning for something I had never undergone before. It was my Santa Claus moment. I was making a list and definitely checking it twice. Before my family crawled into the minivan to drive to Cleveland, all my boxes had been checked on the list. All bumps in the road had been dealt with right up to the great Covid debacle of 2020. I was ready to meet the man who would cut me open and sew me up.

When my surgeon walked into the room, we both had the same puzzled look and thought about each other. My doctor was the only one to verbalize it. "You seem a little young to be here."

We chuckled. I was told that the majority of his surgical cases had been postponed for a later date. He would have postponed mine as well, but I had come all the way from Wisconsin. We chatted about the current environment, and I was told that he was still willing to do the surgery the next day if I was willing to have it done. There was no moment of truth for me. I was all in. I have had this surgery hanging over my head for months at this point. The plans have been made. I was ready. With that confirmation, it was time to make some decisions about the surgery. Wait, what?

I had come all this way to see the best in the business about a valve-sparing procedure, but what happens if the surgeon gets in there and the valve can't be saved? You have to plan for everything. Did I want to have a natural tissue valve replacement or a mechanical replacement? Each one has its merits, but at my age, the mechanical valve could reduce the times I had to come back over the years to keep replacing it as opposed to if it were live tissue.

All my planning, all of my research, and I had never once considered the fact that my valve-sparing procedure might not be able to save my valve. Sometimes I believe I might be one of the dumber smart people you will ever meet. I see optional surgical interventions listed on the surgical consent every week at work. Yet I still arrived in my surgeon's office never once considering the option that my surgery might not go exactly as planned. I wrote a document about what to do if I died, but still hadn't thought about it. Apparently logic had left the building.

Surgical options for valve replacement include:

Mechanical valve - This is a long-lasting valve composed of durable materials that can avoid long-term anticoagulation therapy. For the younger heart patient, this type of replacement could also avoid follow up surgical procedures over time if a natural valve developed another problem.

Tissue valve - A natural valve that could be either human or animal donor tissue. These valves often require anticoagulation therapy.

Ross Procedure - A procedure that borrows a healthy valve and repositions it where the damaged aortic valve resides, then replaces the borrowed valve with a new one.

TAVI/TAVR procedure - Transcatheter aortic valve implantation/ transcatheter aortic valve replacement. Smaller incisions and faster recovery times for the patient fitting the requisite criteria.

The procedure chosen by the surgeon will depend on the valve that needs replacement, the severity of patient symptoms, and the risks of surgery. The information on valve surgery and much more can be found on the website for The American Heart Association at heart.org.

I had a root dilation on the top of my aortic valve. This is otherwise known as an aneurysm, or an excessive localized enlargement of an artery caused by a weakening of the artery wall. If the aneurysm continued to grow unchecked, it could pull at the valve and stretch it, creating the tendency for regurgitation. At that point, the damage it causes can change the procedure entirely. Here I was again, realizing that the best-laid plans were a roadmap drawn on a napkin.

My decisions were made, a surgical plan was in place, and consents were signed. I was given a tote bag full of manuals and instructions and numbers to call for my recovery. My fifteen minutes in the surgeon's office were up, and this man had things to do. Thanks to Covid-19, the surgeon had much less to do than usual, but I got the impression he had no idea how to sit still or relax. His body language insisted that if this man wasn't actively progressing his schedule, the time and space continuum might implode. We shook hands and quickly grabbed some alcohol to rub vigorously over the parts that had touched something other than ourselves and subconsciously agreed to never speak of it again. Then he was gone.

As I sit here today, months displaced from my surgery, I have never seen my surgeon again. His scheduling coordinator says they will work hard to ensure I see him at the one-year check-up, though, so there's that. Regardless of whether that meeting happened or not, I sometimes think about the fact that the surgeon who saved my life only met me in person once for fifteen minutes. To this man, those meetings are a dime a dozen. Something he has done a thousand times. For me as the patient, that was fifteen minutes of talking to the surgeon who would stop my heart, fix what was broken, and give me a new lease on the amount of time I get with my family. I remember every moment of that meeting.

After I left the surgeon's meeting, my walk back to the hotel room to hang out with my family was the longest walk of my life. In actuality, it was about two hundred yards. There is the possibility that at some point in your life, you have found your mind wandering aimlessly. Imagine your thoughts as a freight train, barreling down a track with memories flying by. You can only notice them long enough to recall a moment before they are pushed aside by another memory racing by.

When people say that their life has flashed before their eyes or they were moving in slow motion, I think they are referencing times like these. My measured pace back to the hotel room was in slow motion. I was moving at a normal pace, but my mind couldn't focus on a single thing at once. Memories of my children and the day I was married on the beach popped up and disappeared with each step. It might have been stress, fear, or a combination of the two. All I knew was that I wanted to be with my family.

I try to envision myself as a realistic person, which can occasionally appear negative on the outside. An indication of my plain talk personality would be when I told you to make a document outlining everything you wanted to be done posthumously if something was to happen to you. This reality-based train of thought gives you a hint of how many things race through my mind on a normal day. This walk was as if my mind was on amphetamines.

How do you make sure your kids know how much you love them without freaking them out? How do you try to explain to your wife the last checklist of items that you updated online without seeming like you are worried about the surgery? How do you sleep the night before? As with every surgery, and this wasn't my first time, there is worry about the things that are out of your control. I won't bore you with the details of what my family did all night, but it was just food delivered to the room, some online gaming with my kids, and a lot of hugs that my teenage children didn't cringe or shy away from. This night was one of my greatest achievements in calmness. I did my pre-surgical body wash, had some fun with my family, and then tried to memorize every aspect of their faces before I closed my eyes and hoped for rest.

Pre-surgical wash: To try and avoid situations involving surgical wound infections, patients are given a wash to be used before their surgical day. The most common antibacterial used is chlorhexidine gluconate, also known as Hibiclens. Instructions may include a good scrub, clean towels, and even clean sheets the night before. The concept is to remove as many bacteria that naturally occur on a patient's skin before incision. The bacteria that live on the outside of a person's skin and help to keep them healthy can wreak havoc if they find their way into a surgical incision. Do not shave your body before arriving at the hospital for surgery. Any irritated hair follicles or abrasions can provide an area for bacteria to thrive, and increase your chance for infection.

Chapter 6
Surgery Day

This will be the start of a section that can be viewed by some readers as far too much detail, while it might not be enough for others. I will discuss what happened to me on the way to surgery, but I will also discuss a few things that happen while you are asleep. If this is the type of thing that isn't your cup of tea, feel free to skip right over this and move on to a less descriptive chapter. There is nothing I will discuss that you couldn't readily find in greater detail with a quick online search. If you have been trying to avoid it, I don't want to be the one to ruin it for you now.

You're still here? Last chance to skip ahead. You can always dog-ear this chapter and come back to it later. I have to assume that if you are still reading that you want to hear some of the specifics about surgery day. Either you are the type of person who wants all the details about what is happening to your body, or you just have a morbid curiosity about anatomy and surgery. Whichever one it is, let's talk about the big day and what you can expect.

Surgery day is a busy day at the hospital. It's not as busy for you as it is for everyone else. I arrived early in the morning because I had the first surgery of the day. I liked being first on the schedule because it meant my wife wouldn't be waiting all day for me to go into surgery and then start the process of counting the minutes until it was over. The earlier it starts, the earlier it ends.

By six a.m., I was already in the preoperative waiting area, stripping down to butt naked and wiping down my body with antibacterial cleansing wipes. You will be told that these wipes are meant to cleanse your body of bacteria present on the skin, but the nurse might not mention these wipes will turn you into a sheet of human flypaper. Every surface will be sticky when you are done. Be careful wiping too thoroughly in any hairy areas. I am thinking specifically of in between your cheeky areas. No one wants to try and reposition in a hospital bed while wearing a gown that is too small only to find out your ass hair is being removed by the sheets thanks to a pseudo-glue substance you caked in your crack.

Depending on the supplier at your facility of choice, your gown could be made of paper or a sandpaper-like material. It could be made of very soft material, yet sized for a large child. Some facilities even have gowns made with ports for heaters to keep you warm before you are whisked away to the operating room. Don't worry too much about your attire. Whatever the makeup of the gown is, you won't have to wear it that long.

When you are done getting yourself scrubbed up with a light pine tar marketed as soap and finally get the gown pulled down far enough to cover a portion of your nether region, a wonderful staff member will show up with a smile and an electric razor. This person will then ask you to pull your gown down so they can shave the surgical site. You will hear the phrase "we will keep you covered" a lot in the hospital. They will try. They will fail. You might be a little embarrassed at first. Don't be; this is all part of the process. That process is preparing you for surgery, not your crippling embarrassment.

These people have seen it all. They have seen so many body parts that it doesn't even register on their list of what happened at work that day. In the six months before my heart surgery, I had to have an emergency appendectomy after work one day. I had this procedure at the very same operating suites where I converse with a host of colleagues every day of every week. There isn't a person that was in the room that day who doesn't know exactly how small my penis is. They might giggle when they see me, but no one mentions it.

One thing to remember if you are still nervous about exposing your body to strangers is that this is preoperative preparation. This is not a speed dating luncheon at the country club. You didn't come to the hospital to pick up a young, beautiful nurse. You came to fix your heart. There will be patients in every room having the exact same scenario play out all day long normally. You should put this out of your mind and not give it another thought.

What exactly is the surgical site they need to shave? Well, one would guess correctly that in preparation for a heart surgery it involves shaving the chest. Maybe you are a female and your chest is not hairy. Maybe it is. I'm not here to judge. If there is hair on your chest, that hair needs to go.

Also, depending on what type of procedure you are having, the nurse might need to go a little lower. How low? Like to your ankles low. Vein harvests come from your legs. This is the vein that would be reinserted if you are having a coronary artery bypass graft (CABG). If a surgeon would need access to a groin for a line placement or you are scheduled for an abdominal aortic aneurysm (AAA) repair, then your legs will need to be shaved and prepped as well when you make it to the operating room. All I am saying is that when a nurse tells you they have arrived to shave you, don't be alarmed by the area they start shaving.

For the men, when a washcloth is placed on your penis to shave closer to your manhood than you have probably ever considered, just know that it will be repositioned and the other side is coming next. It's not a ploy to torment you, and there are no hidden camera shows. This is the beginning of a long day for everyone. I will reiterate to try and relax while allowing each professional you come into contact with that day to do their job.

Another common component of preparing patients for surgery involves testing them for bacteria that can complicate stays or lead to an increased chance of hospital-associated infections. These are infections that might result from a procedure that occurred during your stay at the facility. Common causes of infections can be related to IVs, Foley catheters, and breathing tubes. Any situation where a foreign object is entering the body can introduce bacteria into the system.

The most common bacteria associated with these types of infections is Staphylococcus aureus. According to the Centers for Disease Control and Prevention, 30% of adults are colonized with this bacteria, and it is most often found in a patient's nose. In an effort to reduce the risk of infection, all patients are screened preoperatively. A nasal swab will be placed in your nose while in the preoperative area. When the nurse comes at your nose with a swab and you are wondering what a long-stemmed cotton swab has to do with your heart, you can relax and let them scrub your nasal membranes until your eyes water, knowing it is for your safety during the recovery period.

Now that you are nasal swabbed and are left with only the hair on your head and that sticky clump between your cheeks, it is time to move on to something more fun. I use that term lightly. It is similar to describing a car wreck as exhilarating. The next step can be location dependent. At the facility where I work, some anesthesiologists prefer to place all of their own arterial lines and IVs for heart surgery. Other facilities, like the one I went to for my surgery, will roll you into the operating room with no lines inserted and place them all once you are on the table. Granted, I was only awake for the one IV, and someone else might be awake for two, but everyone having heart surgery will wake up with more.

You will hear talk about intravenous lines while you are lying there in pre-op planning to make a break for it. A quick rundown of what the lines are and what you might hear will follow. Plus, we can talk about the additional lines you will wake up with, in case you didn't hear about them beforehand.

A simple intravenous line (IV) can be placed in many different areas on your body. Depending on how difficult your veins are to find or place a catheter into will determine if you get a smaller bore IV to start and a larger one once you are asleep. Occasionally, people can be considered difficult sticks and need to have an ultrasound or a bit of digging to get the gauge (size) of IV that will be necessary to facilitate adequate access to your vasculature while you are having a large surgery. If one of the intravenous lines were to fail in surgery, providers like to have another one at the ready. In a situation where large volumes of fluid are needed due to blood loss, more lines are better. This surgery involves your heart, so blood loss can happen.

Some of these IVs are not small and can pinch a bit, so many providers prefer to let you be asleep for the placement of the line. Other providers might use a local anesthetic to numb the area prior to insertion. It might sound ridiculous at this point, but the initial intravenous line might be the hardest part of the morning heading into surgery. I don't say that to scare you. I say that to put your mind at ease. Most people have managed to get an IV placed at some point in their life. If you can manage that on surgery day, your team will take care of everything else.

The size of the intravenous catheter placed is important for flow. Thanks to a guy named Poiseuille, we know that doubling the size of an IV catheter increases the flow rate by sixteen fold. If you want to get fluids in fast, you want a large catheter to do it. Getting large IVs is similar to buying a brand new car when your old ride has been breaking down. You want the security of the new one, but no one likes paying for it. These peripheral IVs are commonly placed in the arms, but I don't know what your veins look like. The provider who is gaining access will have done this many times before and have a fantastic idea of what you need for the best results.

Another line you will receive will be an arterial line. This line is exactly what it sounds like. While the large gauge IVs mentioned before were placed in a vein with the venous flow, this line will be placed into an artery with the arterial flow. The arterial line is different because it can monitor your blood pressure on a beat-to-beat basis. The contraction of your heart results in rhythmic and pulsatile pressure throughout your body. This line is important because it gives your provider an on-the-spot analysis of what is happening in a patient's body during the surgery. This line will also be needed during heart surgery because the pulsatile flow that is registered by a blood pressure cuff goes away when a patient is on the heart-lung bypass machine (more on this later).

Additionally, blood draws can be taken from arterial lines without the need to poke a patient over and over. Most commonly you will find this line placed in the radial artery of your wrist, but there are no guarantees. Those arteries might be crustier than a Wisconsin fish fry, so your provider could move north to a brachial artery or even place them femoral in your thigh area. Each location has its benefits and detriments. Some locations are less than ideal due to surgical access complications. But if we were dealing with ideal situations, would we be talking about open-heart surgery?

The last line I will mention will be a central line. Again, no one is trying to throw you off with the naming of this particular line. Central venous catheters come in all shapes and sizes. What type of central venous catheter is used might come down to anesthesia preference, as well as the surgeon's preference for postoperative care. There are Swan-Ganz catheters that can be placed through a central line to measure the pulmonary wedge pressure in your heart. There are monitors for central venous pressure to assess the fluid dynamics of patients. There are many types of catheters with specific purposes to help providers take care of patients.

A patient can get a longer, large gauge line placed with multiple ports that can stay in for extended periods to avoid things like medicines that may cause irritation if given peripherally.

Central lines also avoid multiple sticks as smaller peripheral IVs will age out and need to be replaced more quickly based on facility policy to avoid infections. The applications for these types of central venous catheters can range from chemotherapy, dialysis, blood tests, and medicine and fluid administration in heart surgery.

You will commonly find this central venous catheter placed on the right side of your neck when you wake up. The most common placement for this type of line is in the right internal jugular vein. This vein provides a great combination of safety and ease of access for the person putting it in. When you wake up from surgery, there will be nurses and staff making sure you keep your hands away from this catheter. It is stitched into your skin and covered to keep it clean. You don't want this line getting an infection, and you certainly don't want to pull it out. The exact detailed instructions you will probably receive are "don't touch it."

A half-hour into my morning, I was clean and prepped for surgery. A transport person rolled my bed up to the door outside of the operating room where I met the anesthesiologist who was overseeing my case. This doctor was the same man who had talked to the surgeon on my behalf and gotten me scheduled as the first case of the day. This anesthesiologist had worked with a couple of guys who are currently in my group back home. Each person I spoke with had wonderful things to say about him. These things were all true.

This anesthesiologist was an extremely nice guy and very personable. Anesthesia professionals are very knowledgeable and are happy to fill in any gaps that you might still have pertaining to the anesthetic for your case. I didn't have many questions myself, but this would be where you get some last-minute explanations about what happens with anesthesia if you still aren't sure. I also met a certified registered nurse anesthetist (CRNA) who would be taking care of me as well during my case. These are advanced practice nurses who specialize in anesthesia after undergoing a multi-year degree program following nursing school and usually several years working in a critical care environment.

It was an odd feeling for me rolling into an operating room on the bed instead of pushing it. As we entered the operating room, everyone introduced themselves, and I moved myself onto the cold operating room table. With my permission, a coworker had mentioned my surgery in an anesthesia forum that many professionals frequent. My colleague requested that any anesthesia friends who might be working that day should look for me in surgery. A simple request from one anesthesia provider to another.

Since most cases in the hospital had been canceled, I think I recall at least four CRNAs introducing themselves to me. Each person in the operating room took a moment to introduce themselves and tell me their role. Every single person you will see in the operating room is there for you. You are not a bother. You are the reason that each person came into work that day. It might be scary seeing all the unfamiliar equipment in the operating room. Rest assured, every professional that you meet is part of a dedicated team who is there to protect you and make sure you get the best possible outcome. It might be your first time in surgery, but normally these providers have done this procedure thousands of times before. There was an IV poke in my hand, and that was the last thing I remember about the operating room.

What happened to me while I was asleep? The specifics of your surgery could differ from mine based on what type of procedure you are having. I had a valve-sparing procedure to replace the ascending aorta and preserve the natural aortic valve. The actual particulars for my procedure are that the surgeon will cut the aorta above the aortic valve annulus and the coronary ostia. These are the openings where the coronary arteries are attached to the aortic root. This will begin the removal of the aneurysm to be replaced with a synthetic graft.

What did I just say? That is exactly why my goal here isn't to delve too deeply into what occurs in each procedure. If you have questions about the specifics of your particular surgery, I would encourage you to ask your surgeon to explain what is going to happen. Even if you search it on the internet, you might find subtle variations listed. Or you might find that the descriptions could be overly vague as well. Each surgeon has their own technique that could be somewhat different from what you find. Never be afraid to ask questions. You will not be wasting their time. They want you to understand what is going to happen once in the operating room.

These people are surgeons, not magicians. There is no benefit in maintaining a mystic aura about the operating room. A standard procedure in cardiac surgeons' offices is that once you are told the necessary procedure, a brochure describing the surgery will be available to help you understand the process. If you don't like the information the brochure has, the internet will have numerous resources to assist you. Most heart hospitals have fairly descriptive web presences available if you search for your procedure. I used the website of my hospital, and any other website I could find, and then I went into my Clinical Anesthesiology textbook from school.

The next clarification we should make is about all these doctors you are seeing. What is the difference between the heart doctor from the clinic and the heart doctor in the operating room? Think of cardiac doctors as two separate classifications of physicians. A cardiologist that sees you about your rhythm, rate, and the general health of your heart is like the electrician version of the cardiac world. This doctor is looking at electrical impulses and lines of connection throughout the process of your heartbeat. The cardiologist can do testing to determine the health and history of the cardiovascular system.

The cardiac surgeon who cracks you and rebuilds your pipes is the plumber of the cardiac world. In my case, the surgeon was replacing one big ass pipe. There are additional arteries at the arch of the aorta called the great vessels. These are smaller pipes that still hold a very important function in the plumbing of your vasculature. Think of the main water line to your house and all the different lines to each bathroom. A bathroom leak is more manageable than if someone breaks the largest water line with the greatest pressure right in the middle of your yard.

My surgeon's goal was to replace this huge mainline pipe before it burst. This would, in turn, save the aortic valve below it. If an aneurysm is left to grow, it can eventually pull and manipulate the valve below it. This causes additional problems and changes the type of procedure that will have to be done. An ancillary benefit of having my procedure electively before a rupture or dissection of the aorta was avoiding the high likelihood of dying. I am all for that.

Another very common procedure that you will hear a lot is a coronary artery bypass graft, or CABG (pronounced cabbage). This is where your *plumber* physician will harvest veins, most commonly from your legs, and replace the arteries on your heart to repair a blockage. You may need to go on cardiopulmonary bypass (CPB) to have this done. However, some institutions now perform off-pump coronary artery bypass (OPCAB). The end destinations are the same, but the route to get there is different.

All of these terms and letters will mean very little to you unless you know that you are having that procedure in particular. The variations might seem subtle, but completely shape the experience you will have in the operating room. While you might have a very different procedure while on the table than what I had, the recovery and preparation will be similar to my own and the millions of people who have had surgery before you. Some people bond over hobbies or sports, but we will all be a family sharing a common scar soon enough.

Before your surgical day, a procedure called a cardiac catheterization will be done to determine if there are problems with arterial flow and vessel blockage in the heart. This procedure will happen in the cardiac catheterization lab. The cath lab is a type of procedure room where patients can be tested under fluoroscopy to determine the frequency and severity of vessel blockage as well as any other procedure that requires direct visualization. This is usually a workup done for your cardiac surgeon but not by your cardiac surgeon.

This procedure will determine if and how many vessels need to be repaired due to blockage. A heart catheterization is a process where an IV catheter is most commonly placed in your wrist, and contrast dye is infused under fluoroscopy to evaluate the flow through these cardiac vessels. A lack of flow or blockage could be the reason for your surgery. It could also be something that needs to be repaired when an even larger issue is being replaced on your heart. These arteries are checked prior to surgery because there is no need for a new faucet if the water doesn't turn on.

The list of possible procedures can get quite extensive. There are valve replacements, vessel replacements of all shapes and sizes, and even complete transplants. So while the actual procedure can vary, there are a few things that we all can share during this time. The first thing that we share is the types of lines they use to make sure patients are monitored appropriately. If you are having a vessel or a valve replaced, the lines are something that we can all count on having at the end.

The next item we all share might be one of the most feared things involved in this process. That elephant in the room would be the sternotomy. A sternotomy is classified as an incision into the sternum. That seems like an oversimplification of the process, as it will involve a bone saw after a skin incision exposes your sternum. Have you ever heard the term simple truths? I have heard more people ask about this than have actually asked what type of surgery I had done.

There are a few reasons that patients might not hear about the actual sternotomy that will happen during their procedure. If you are married and your spouse's greatest cooking skill is burning water, what do you say when they ask you if they are a good cook? The simple truth can be scary and occasionally hurtful. However, this chapter is about the reality of the surgery. Certain procedures require the exposure of your heart to the surgeon, hence the term open-heart surgery. That is where the sternotomy comes in.

How bad will this be? Cutting through my sternum with a saw is super scary! I am certain that the bony plate is there for a reason, and using a bone saw to dismantle it seems like a big deal! The reality of the situation is this process is less risky than the rest of your procedure. And it won't be scary for you at all. You are asleep. The only reason we are talking about this is that it will come up later in the recovery portion of this story.

Once the sternotomy has been done, there will be an instrument placed in the incision that spreads the two sides apart. This instrument is used to make a little room to work in your chest cavity. It's just easier to fix a leak under the sink if you get the cleaning supplies out of the way and shine a light under there. When the expansion takes place, it will spread your ribs away from their natural position. This will cause your ribs to create pressure on your spine and back muscles because it forces them into an unnatural position. This is not as dangerous as it sounds. However, it does lead to sore muscles after surgery.

Unfortunately, this is a necessary component of your surgery. It will be painful when you are recovering because of the soreness it can cause in your back. You might be worried about how your chest feels after having a sternotomy. In my experience, the muscles in my back suffered far greater soreness than my chest incision ever did. Do not be afraid of the sternotomy. It is just a scary prelude to a greater story that is being written for you.

There are too many variables for me to talk about the specifics of what each surgeon prefers, techniques, or even all the different types of open-heart procedures that can be done. Advancing techniques change the landscape of what is possible in healthcare constantly. Valve replacements can now be done through small incisions that minimize recovery times. It is an exciting time in surgery, but nothing that you need to hear anything additional about for this chapter. Any questions you have for your specific surgery should be directed to your surgeon and the literature provided by the facility.

Chapter 7
While You Were Sleeping

What happens to your body once the drugs set in while you are in the operating room? Do you care as long as you wake up at the end of the procedure? If you don't care what happens while you are asleep or get squeamish thinking about surgery, then this chapter is another waste of time. I will take a moment to discuss in general terms some of the things that will happen to your body while you are asleep to make it somewhat easier to understand why certain things happen in recovery. Again, these are likely scenarios, not certainties. My disclaimer is still the same. Every surgeon and surgery carries with it a very detailed process that is individualized for staff and patients.

One of the larger events in open-heart surgery that will affect your body postoperatively will be cardiopulmonary bypass (CPB). This is a process that will divert venous blood away from the heart, add oxygen and remove carbon dioxide, and then return the blood to the body through a large artery. A common artery that is used for many surgeries during this process is the aorta.

What does any of that even mean? It means that almost all blood flow through the heart and a majority of the flow through the lungs stops during surgery while on cardiopulmonary bypass. A complex machine with its own operator, known as a perfusionist, will provide artificial perfusion and ventilation while you are on bypass during your procedure. The actual name of this device is the Heart-Lung Machine. That is the truth. You can look it up. It is like medical terminology got to a point where someone said, "I'm done thinking of complicated names."

I won't go into the intricacies of this machine, but it has all the capabilities of what your body can do in regards to a reservoir of blood, oxygenator, and even a heat exchanger. It takes a machine the size of a Harley Davidson with a person trained solely to run it to mimic what your heart and lungs do. Think about that for a minute. If you can get past the scary part of this surgery happening to you, it is a modern feat of technology that is downright miraculous. The fact that you are having heart surgery today as opposed to fifty years ago means that you will have access to numerous miracles of modern medicine.

While an ingenious machine, there is a downside to cardiopulmonary bypass. This technique is non-physiological. Bypass is classified as non-physiologic because arterial pressure is typically below average, and blood flow is nonpulsatile. What exactly does that mean? Try to envision that your heart in all of its complicated structure is a pump. Imagine that every time your heart squeezes, a rush of blood gets pushed forward in your vasculature. Your blood pressure will be high on the squeeze while it quickly flows from your heart and fills your aorta, then diminishes momentarily for the refilling of your heart chambers. These numbers are what will be translated into systolic and diastolic when your blood pressure is taken.

The heart-lung machine might be able to apply oxygen and filter contaminants, but there would be no benefit to having it shoot blood back into the body at varying degrees of pressure. Your blood becomes a constant flow at a measured pace back into your body. This is the nature of cardiopulmonary bypass being non-physiologic.

Is this process damaging to your body? It is less damaging than the surgeon asking an assistant to put his finger in your heart like the little Dutch boy while he works. The process of cardiopulmonary bypass should be described as stressful to your body. A stressful necessity I might add in a lot of surgeries. To mitigate some of the stress the organs might receive while on bypass, systemic hypothermia is usually initiated.

That means the surgeon will drop your body temperature down to around 20-32°C (That is 68-89°F in freedom units).

The reason for cooling a patient can be associated with the van't Hoff equation that theorizes metabolic oxygen requirements are cut in half for every 10°C reduction in body temperature. On occasion, other methods of cooling might include topical hypothermia involving an ice slush or cardioplegia, which is a chemical solution for arresting myocardial electrical activity. These methods are all employed to protect your heart and other organs while your system is being stressed on cardiopulmonary bypass during surgery.

Once you are asleep, how will they keep an eye on your heart before it is exposed? A monitor that will be employed during surgery that can lead to a bit of throat discomfort during recovery is transesophageal echocardiography (TEE). TEE can provide a real-time analysis with valuable information about cardiac anatomy and function during surgery before a patient is on bypass.

A TEE can be used to detect ventricular abnormalities, the dimensions of the heart chambers, valve anatomy, and even the presence of air in the heart. The TEE can be used to confirm the cannulation of the coronary sinus for the surgeon as well. This is another invaluable tool for the surgical team as it provides an instant roadmap that is always current as work is being started during the surgery.

Why in the world would this monitor cause throat pain? For those unfamiliar with what a TEE probe looks like, it is a long flexible tube that is placed into the esophagus to provide images to a screen from below the heart. These images are created by using ultrasound to develop a moving image. Unfortunately, this technology comes at the price of shoving a small garden hose down your throat. Not literally a garden hose, but you get the idea.

Once placed in the esophagus, the probe will be spun around, pushed in, pulled back, and pushed in again. I am only trying to convey that while an important part of your surgery, this device can cause some soreness when all is said and done. But if you are holding throat discomfort in one hand and a lack of images and measurements during heart surgery in the other, I am picking the sore throat every time.

While you are in surgery, another treatment that can affect your body postoperatively is anticoagulation therapy. This means medicating your system with heparin to avoid blood clots forming in the heart-lung machine and creating problems during cardiopulmonary bypass. Valvular surgeries have a higher risk of blood clot formation, and anticoagulation can help to avoid that from occurring intraoperatively. Blood clots can lead to strokes, and I haven't read any literature where a stroke improved a heart surgery outcome.

Heparin is a naturally occurring glycosaminoglycan used as a blood thinner in surgeries. A blood test is performed regularly throughout the surgery to ensure the heparin dose keeps your blood anticoagulated at an appropriate level during the procedure. While the administration of heparin can increase the risk of bleeding, its benefits far outweigh the risks in heart surgery.

This test to determine anticoagulation levels is called the Activated Clotting Time (ACT) test. This test will determine the amount of time it takes for your blood to form a clot. Once the surgery reaches a certain point and anticoagulation is no longer needed, a reversal agent called protamine sulfate will be administered. Protamine will be administered over five minutes, and it binds to the heparin and forms a stable ion pair that can be broken down by the body's natural reticuloendothelial system. Wow, that's a mouthful. It means one drug binds to the other drug and makes the anticoagulation mechanism of the heparin stop working. Just like that, your blood can form a clot in a normal amount of time again.

Why do I mention anticoagulation therapy at all? Once you are awake and assessing your body, it looks eerily similar to a beating instead of surgery. What happened to you? Lots of medications will be given during your surgery, but this drug, in particular, will often leave you a parting gift of bruises in recovery.

The main reason for those bruises is that during this period of anticoagulation, every part of your body that has a line placed, an incision made, or a chest tube inserted will bruise very easily. When your blood has trouble clotting, your body keeps sending more blood to the area to try anyway. These extra red blood cells being filled into the tissue will become the beautiful purple areas you see when you wake up. Body parts that are weighty and don't move for a certain period might see some blood pooling as well.

After a couple of days postoperatively, you will start to look more like a car wreck survivor than a surgical patient. Bruises take time to recover and depending on your tendency to bruise before the anticoagulation therapy, it could be jarring for people to see. There could be some soreness associated with some of the larger areas, but it will all pass in time. Just don't be alarmed that it looked like surgery was conducted with a baseball bat and a pair of brass knuckles. This therapy was done for your safety during surgery, not your comfort during recovery.

Once the surgeon has done his repair, you should be off the table in about fifteen minutes, right? For some reason, most patients stay focused on their schedule even when it becomes something completely out of their control. People get very concerned about the time frame of surgery. If you aren't the first case of the day, more often than not there can be delays in your actual surgical time.

Don't get upset. When a patient is visibly bothered that they were supposed to go into surgery at noon, and it is now two hours later, we try to explain that surgical estimates are just that, estimates. Some things can happen faster, and other things can take more time. I have seen patients so upset that they had to wait that they left the hospital and didn't have surgery at all that day. Never a heart surgery, but smaller cases involving orthopedics or elective procedures.

Think about that for a moment. You have done all the appointments necessary to have surgery. You already got the insurance approval done and made the date. You washed your body and didn't eat all day, waiting for your turn. However, because a surgeon took their time with another patient, you storm off and skip a surgery you know you need and want.

It might seem wild, but it happens. All the staff in the operating room are working as hard as they can, and then to be yelled at because they were taking care of another patient can be difficult to hear. When families ask me how long a procedure will take, I normally say, "until it's done right." If a patient yells at me because we are behind schedule, they never look pleased when I ask if I should talk to the surgeon about making up some time on their case. Be patient and stay calm. Ask for drugs if deep breathing isn't working for you. This is your life, not a track meet.

A lot of work has gone into getting you to the operating room. Even more has happened once the surgeon has made the repair. Now that he is done, a lot more still needs to happen. If you were on cardiopulmonary bypass and your body is cooled, it will need to be rewarmed. If there was a vein taken from your leg, there might be an incision down there spanning two feet, or there may be a small port incision used for scope insertion.

Every incision will need to be sewn and covered and wrapped, as well as the one on your chest. That midline incision is not a couple of stitches and you are good either. You could have wires placed to hold everything together nice and tight, or possibly a metal plate placed for larger people. Then there are sutures and dressings. The chest tubes will need to be sewn in and covered as well. There is an entire team working to make sure that you are put together securely. The point of all this is to say don't worry about the time frame. This is your body. There are no shortcuts.

Lastly, you are asleep. The entire surgery will pass in the blink of an eye. If you are worried about your family and the time they will be waiting, don't bother. If you have a family member that you are certain will be aggravated at the time it takes for a surgeon to repair your heart, ask them to stay home. That isn't a person that will be helpful with your recovery anyway. This process is about you and no one else.

Your operation is the single most important thing that will be happening in your life that day. Because of this operation, you have been granted the gift of more days. Those days equal more time with your loved ones. Relax as much as you can. Enjoy the moments with the people who are closest to you if they can join you. You should know that a dedicated team will take every moment necessary to give you the best outcome possible. Surround yourself with people who will be supportive and attentive to your needs. Your surgical staff will take care of everything else.

Chapter 8

How Asleep Is Asleep

A question that people in the anesthesia community get quite a bit is how do we, as providers, know the patient will be asleep? Additionally, a common statement heard is that the patient or someone they knew woke up during anesthesia. These types of statements can create a fear that the patient might suddenly wake up while this massive procedure is going on in their chest. This chapter is meant to allay some of those fears.

I promise this section will be kept to a minimum because I am not biased toward anesthesia in the slightest little bit (sarcasm added). We will discuss a few items pertaining to the gas passers in the operating room so you understand what these providers are talking about when you hear some of the terminology. It will help to have a better grasp of what exactly will occur once you crawl onto that operating room table.

First, let's address what your anesthesia professional will be doing while you are in the operating room. Anesthesia is the management of pain and consciousness from a central nervous system perspective. That statement might sound a bit broad and non-specific. Anesthesia is a fairly broad term as well. That term can cover a whole host of different techniques and methods to accomplish a single goal: your safety and comfort as a patient.

Anesthesia can be described as the pasta noodle of the medical world. You can say pasta, and it could mean spaghetti, rigatoni, macaroni, fettucini, or any number of other types of noodles. They are all pasta but can vary in subtle ways. It is more of a catch-all when an anesthesia professional says you will be under anesthesia for surgery. There are many varieties of anesthesia, but those numbers are reduced to a single category when you are having open heart surgery. That category is general anesthesia.

Various types of anesthesia include spinal anesthesia, monitored anesthesia care, and general anesthesia. Even within each of these types, there are multiple ways to achieve success with varying drugs and combinations of different techniques. For open heart surgery, patients will be under general anesthesia, whereby they will be completely and totally asleep.

A spinal anesthetic is most commonly used for lower body procedures involving procedures that would require a patient to not feel anything below a specific level of the spinal cord. That is where a local anesthetic would be applied to the corresponding area of the spinal nerves. A local anesthetic is similar in the manner it blocks nerve pathways so the patient doesn't feel pain at the surgical site.

A local block just involves a more specific area than the spinal, which will block everything below a certain level of the spinal cord. If a patient needs their foot operated on, then local could be applied to the foot and ankle. A local anesthetic is what a patient would receive in their arm before a big IV if they were going to be awake while they did it. A spinal would numb a larger regional area in cases involving things like total knee arthroplasty or a C-section.

Monitored anesthesia care, commonly referred to as MAC anesthesia, is a sedation anesthetic. This means the patient will be breathing on their own without the assistance of a breathing device for the duration of the case. MAC is often combined with a local anesthetic to improve comfort. When someone says they "woke up" during anesthesia, this is what they are referring to in terms of the anesthetic used during their procedure.

MAC anesthesia is like a big nap. Patients can technically still hear things in the room like conversations and work being done. Depending on if a patient obstructs when they sleep, they might not be kept as deeply asleep to try and prevent that obstruction from happening. The most common drug for achieving this type of anesthesia is Propofol. This was the drug of choice for a certain pop star and is what a lot of people associate it with. In the anesthesia world, it can be known as the milk of amnesia.

General anesthesia is the fully-asleep, down-for-the-count, no-questions-asked anesthesia. This is the anesthetic where a patient will be in a profound state of sleep and completely unarousable. During your open heart procedure, a patient will get an endotracheal tube placed past the vocal cords with a balloon inflated to protect the airway. The process of intubation uses a mini pickaxe-looking device called a laryngoscope.

This tool allows the anesthesia provider to visualize the airway and vocal cords for proper placement of the endotracheal tube. When a patient asks how I know they will be asleep before the intubation, I inform them that a weight-based calculation of induction anesthetics will be administered, and a lash reflex tested before we proceed. In reality, if patients weren't asleep when intubation started, then I would get my fingers bitten quite a bit.

Patients in open heart surgery will receive an endotracheal tube because they will be placed on a ventilator that does the breathing for them while in surgery. This process is called intubation. An endotracheal tube is a component that serves several purposes during your surgery. It allows a patient's airway to be protected and supplies a means to ventilate them. The endotracheal tube is a pliable material that can irritate your throat when you wake up from surgery on occasion. Some people will complain of a sore throat for a day or so after their procedure due to the irritation from the endotracheal tube.

How your anesthesia provider handles this irritating scenario is specific to their practice style. When I had my appendectomy, an old friend of mine was taking care of my anesthetic. He didn't want me to have sore vocal cords when I woke up, so he used a device to spray a local anesthetic into the back of my throat. The device is called a Laryngotracheal Topicalization Anesthesia (LTA) kit, and it has a disposable syringe and cannula. A provider will place the black line on the LTA device at the glottis, squeeze local anesthetic onto the area, and no more sore throat.

When I woke up from my appendectomy, I thought I was choking because of the numbness in my throat and my vocal cords. I coughed for an hour after surgery. That process has been successful for my friend and other patients numerous times before. Yet my experience was less than satisfactory. I am using this as an example to reiterate that practices vary, as do patient responses. This provider did nothing wrong. This technique is effective and helpful. It just didn't work for me personally. You have to remember this scenario when hearing or reading about other people's experiences. There will be some techniques that might possibly work differently for you than they did for others, sometimes better or sometimes worse.

What type of drugs will be used to induce anesthesia? Common drugs include amnestics, paralytics, anxiolytics, and narcotics. Within each class of these drugs, there are many options. The specifics of what is chosen are up to the preference of the anesthesia provider and historical data for the patient. Every bartender has a drink he likes to mix. I am happy to make up a statistic and say Propofol is used 99% of the time as an induction agent. If a recipe calls for salt and you have some Morton's in the cabinet, what do you use for an alternative? Nothing! You use salt. It's easy; it's right on the shelf, and you know it will work.

I am trying to keep this chapter as simple as possible for people that might have a question about drugs. It's not Pharmacology 101, and this is about as far as you will ever get from a textbook. I will not be including the semi-confusing descriptions of drug mechanisms of action for those that are interested in the pharmacokinetics involved. If you care about that type of thing, these descriptions will not be satisfactory to you. It won't hurt my feelings if you want to look them up.

The only thing you need to know about Propofol is it might burn when it is injected. Some local anesthetic might be injected first through the IV to reduce the burning. It might help. It might not. I have seen a broad spectrum of responses to how badly Propofol burns when it is administered. I have seen grandmothers who don't bat an eye to young, strapping weightlifters who scream and yell when it hits their veins. The good news? You probably won't remember either way. Propofol's mechanism of action creates a rapid time to onset of unconsciousness, normally 15-30 seconds, due to rapid distribution from plasma to the CNS.

The paralytics used in surgery are to make sure you don't move while the big fix is underway. There was a movie several years back with a man who was having a heart procedure that had anesthetic awareness. He was paralyzed, but his mind was completely awake. This movie was fiction. It was supposed to be a suspenseful drama, but for medical professionals, it more closely resembled a comedy. There won't be drunk people and dimly lit operating rooms either. Patients should not confuse entertainment and conjecture for fact and reality. You will not be lying in the operating room having an internal monologue during your procedure.

Anxiolytics, commonly benzodiazepines, are used to relax patients and make them forget most of the morning before surgery. These drugs are commonly administered by IV in adults. There are varying degrees of these types of drugs. Many people have had an anxiolytic at some point in their life. A common preoperative anxiolytic is midazolam. Characteristics like your age, size, and whether or not you are climbing the walls can help determine an appropriate dose of anxiety medicine as well. You can play it cool if you like. Surgery is a big deal for most people. If you are nervous, it doesn't make you appear weak to anyone to ask for a little something to take the edge off.

Narcotics, most commonly known as opioids, are for pain control. Perhaps you have heard that there is an epidemic going on regarding narcotics. Maybe it is a personal stance on why you do not want them. This is the one drug class that you need to be honest with your providers about regarding how you would like it handled.

There are adjunct therapies that can help minimize the amount of narcotics taken during and after surgery. Some patients respond better to adjuncts than others. Opioids can affect respiratory rates and blood pressure. Your personal medical history will dictate what type and amount of opioids that are best for you. I was not personally opposed to having something that works as effectively and as quickly as opioids used for my surgery. That personal opinion would change postoperatively, and we will discuss that later.

If you have any additional questions or concerns about pharmacokinetics or ventilator settings, your anesthesia provider is a great person to ask. This person will be watching over your every breath and heartbeat for your entire surgery. Before and after the surgeon has come and gone, your anesthesia provider will be with you. If you ever meet a dashingly handsome anesthesia provider with a terrible southern accent while in Wisconsin, ask if he knows me. If he is average-looking and asks if you are nervous and then tells you he is too, it's just a joke to relieve the tension. Say hello and we can chat.

Chapter 9
I'm Awake

As my eyes fluttered open after surgery, I started to notice things in the room. I had no idea how long I had been awake without actually being aware of it. One of my greatest fears with having surgery would be the unfortunate scenario that I might wake up still intubated. There was nothing about the surgery that scared me more than waking up with an endotracheal tube still in place. Some people might consider this much less scary than some other things we have already discussed, but not me.

This fear might be considered irrational. Well, I am also afraid of spiders. Even the little ones. That isn't rational either. I can just smash a spider with my foot if I have to. Still, I won't be going to a pet store to bring home a tarantula anytime soon. Fears are fears, irrational or not. Here I was, lying in a bed with my wrists secured by straps to the side rails and an endotracheal tube in my airway. Not my favorite memory.

When you wake up from surgery, your gag reflex has returned. It isn't so much that you can't breathe, but more of a panicking sensation that you can't breathe as easily. Imagine trying to suck in a huge breath through a large straw. Seems a bit scary, doesn't it? Naturally, I started to motion to the nurses and pointed toward the endotracheal tube. I remember a younger nurse coming over and telling me that I wasn't ready for the tube to come out yet. I watched her walk away and return a few moments later with a syringe of medicine that she pushed into a port in my IV. Slowly I started to drift back off to sleep, caring less and less about my breathing. At least there weren't any spiders that I could see.

Logically, one could assume that when I woke up the second time that my respirations had grown stronger and the endotracheal tube was gone. If that was your guess, you would be wrong. My greatest surgical fear was being lived out a second time. I started to panic a bit with the sensation of the tube still in my airway. I remember being a bit more frantic this time with my emotions. The response from the staff this time around was that more people came to the bedside to evaluate my respiratory status.

In your mind, an emergency is unfolding. It is not. If I had the time or ability to think and relax, I would have realized that as well. At this point, you are still groggy from an anesthesia-induced nap. You aren't thinking, only reacting to the situation at hand. What seemed like an eternity was only minutes in actuality.

I can only assume that I was pulling adequate tidal volumes at this point in the process. The term for removing an endotracheal tube is extubation. There are standard extubation criteria involving terms such as spontaneous tidal volume and vital capacity. Providers will look at how many liters per minute a patient is breathing and at what level of oxygen support they are receiving. All of these are indicators to assess whether a patient can protect their airway and take large enough breaths to maintain appropriate oxygen saturation. The key is a patient strong enough to keep the endotracheal tube out once it is removed.

At this point, I had met the criteria for the staff to be satisfied I could be extubated successfully. The endotracheal tube's balloon was deflated, and the tube was removed from my airway. The main difference between coughing after many surgeries and coughing after open heart surgery would be the risk of putting too much pressure on the new hardware you just had installed. For all the car folks out there, I would compare hard coughing and vagal maneuvers after heart surgery to pouring a glass of water in the gas tank of your hotrod. It might not do anything, but it never helps.

Extubation is more a question of knowing when the breaking point might be that could cause an issue. Since no one can know that, we want to avoid the situation altogether. Respiratory will want you to be able to pull adequate tidal volumes so you don't struggle once the tube is gone. But the rest of the staff wants you to not fight and cough on it while it's still in place. Like a healthy relationship, there is a give and take that must be employed. Your safety is the determining factor in every decision.

Once my endotracheal tube was out and my hands were untied, the fog in my brain started to slowly lift. This is where the new phase of recovery begins. I had just completed the number one checkmark on every list of every person that has open-heart surgery. It's right at the top, first thing. Don't die! Here I was, alive and slowly starting to realize who I was and where I was.

The room was unfamiliar. I was in the cardiac intensive care unit. People were scurrying around and checking different things now that I am awake and talking. How was my pain? Here is another spoiler alert, I hurt a bit and so will you. One of the handy-dandy devices that were hooked into an IV somewhere on my body was a pain pump. This is a device that loads a syringe or bag of narcotics to an intravenous line that distributes it with the push of a button. The narcotic is picked in an order set by the surgeon or anesthesia. The pump will only allow a certain amount of opioids to be administered over a specific time period no matter how much you hit that button.

The first click of that button was meant to dampen the pain that was radiating from everywhere and nowhere in particular at this point. Do you want to know what is worse than the pain following open-heart surgery? The same level of pain with nausea dumped on top of it. I consider my pain tolerance to be pretty good. Throughout a lifetime of smaller surgeries and injuries, I hadn't taken a lot of narcotics. The narcotics I had received in the past were taken without issue. The bad news for me was this was not going to be like the other times. Even worse news for me, this would be a recurring theme.

My pain pump had fentanyl in it. This opioid has a relatively quick onset. The fentanyl was fast to pain relief and equally fast to vomiting for me. Here I am, just getting my bearings in the cardiac ICU. After the fun memory of the tube coming out of my throat, now I am hurling the bile from my empty stomach into a basin. I can't sit up on my own, so the bed is angled to help me avoid covering myself in vomit. After that quick meal of acid chowder, I was tired and more than happy to sleep for a bit. Oddly enough, when I woke up the pain had not subsided. It was right where I left it. Also, there was the button. Have you ever heard the saying...

Fool me once, shame on you. Fool me twice, shame on me.

This saying is now describing my relationship with fentanyl. It was the same story as the last time. I am chucking up the nothingness that inhabits my stomach yet again. But this time, I have the wherewithal to inform these wonderful nurses to take that button away from me. I will not be using it again.

In the midst of telling me it was going to be okay and wiping my mouth, an idea was born. Let's try another opioid! Oh boy, the excitement was palpable. If I had been given a moment to clear my mind, I might have had the sense to ask for some meperidine to reduce the chance of a third opportunity to perform the call of the walrus. I was not given that moment, and my mind was as clear as trigonometry to my seven-year-old.

Instead, I was given intravenous hydromorphone. I hope you can guess how that went as well. Three strikes and you are out. I was hurting, but the pain was lower on the scale than my irritation with the constant vomiting. Plus the added fear that continuous retching was going to undo my new graft. No more narcotics for me. I had decided that pain control for me would be acetaminophen. I know what you are thinking. You are thinking, this guy can't make it through recovery from open-heart surgery and only take acetaminophen. Wrong. That was exactly how I did it.

I am not telling you this to seem like I am some tough guy. I only mention it because every person is different. Pain is highly subjective. Personally, one of the worst feelings in the world for me is the sensation that I need to throw up and then having to wait around for it. Then the act of hurling is no picnic. Plus, you can imagine that those heavings are not the best thing for a new incision and work done on your heart anyway. How you respond to treatment and the decisions made for pain control will be personal. I would encourage you to use whatever works best and not think about if it is wrong or right. Just decide if it feels wrong or right.

Thus the beginning of my recovery process started a little rocky. This does not mean that this will happen to you when you wake up. You might not have much pain. The pain medicine could fix what is bothering you, or you could hurt and find the pain management difficult to get right. Just prepare yourself mentally for whatever situation you might find yourself in. This surgery will be unlike any other procedure you might have had in the past.

Let's take a quick assessment of what I woke up with after surgery. There was an IV in both arms. The arterial line was added to my left-hand side in my radial artery. Then there was a central line sticking out of my neck on the right side placed in the right internal jugular. All very normal stuff. We talked about these lines. There were no surprises there.

There was also a dressing over my midline incision. You might read about minimally invasive stuff when you are searching online before surgery. That was not what I was looking at. That is not what you will be looking at if you are reading this book for open-heart surgery. My incision was a hint over fourteen inches long. I am a tall enough guy, so it seemed appropriate. I wouldn't want you to get the impression you will be waking up with some three-inch incision on your chest. It's true, the incision will be noticeable in a bikini. But thanks to the incision, you will get more bikini seasons.

A Foley catheter had been placed, which is a catheter tube that runs into your bladder to drain urine so you don't have to struggle to get up to pee. It collects the urine in a bag so nurses can track your output after surgery as well. This can ensure your kidneys are working fine and help to determine if you need medication to relieve some of the extra fluid in your body after surgery. A

Foley catheter is a low-tech monitor that can be vital in the management of your fluid balance postoperatively.

There was a second dressing below the midline incision covering two rubber tubes and some coiled wires that were taped to my abdomen. The rubber tubes are the chest tubes that will be placed to keep fluid from accumulating in your thorax. The chest tubes will be running to the side of your bed and connected to a reservoir. This reservoir allows staff to monitor how much fluid is coming from your chest. Another tube will run from the reservoir to the wall where low intermittent suction will be applied to draw the fluid from your thoracic cavity.

The coiled wires were not hooked up to anything for me, but that is not always the case. These wires that are placed are temporary pacemaker wires. One of the possible side effects of being on cardiac bypass is that when the heart is restarted after the repair, there can be some issues with keeping it in an appropriate rhythm. The goal is to maintain a normal rhythm and not be required to hook those wires to a temporary pacemaker.

Occasionally, the process does not work, and the heart remains in an abnormal rhythm for a time. When this occurs, a temporary pacemaker can be implemented to pace the heart and let things reacclimate over time. The majority of the time, that is all that is needed. There are scenarios where the heart can have trouble staying in a normal rhythm and additional therapy needs to be looked at.

In this situation, antiarrhythmic medication can be applied for some rhythms to see if they can be managed without additional procedures. If antiarrhythmics are not successful, there is the potential that a permanent pacemaker might need to be placed. There is a relatively small chance that this would be the case, but understand that it is still a chance. If a pacemaker is required after your heart surgery, this does not mean something went wrong. It also does not mean that something is still broken in your heart.

These are conduction issues involving pathways in your heart tissues. It involves the flow of impulses from one point to the next. If the pathway is interrupted by something, so is the impulse. People can have issues with rhythm without ever having an issue with their valves or circulation. Some people have heart surgery and no pacemaker. Other people have pacemakers and no heart surgery. Occasionally, some people can have both.

A pacemaker is a small device that can be placed in the chest or abdomen to help control abnormal heart rhythms. This device uses electrical pulses to prompt the heart to beat at a normal rate. Pacemakers can be temporary or permanent and are classified by a five-letter code. This code denotes the chambers paced, chambers sensed, pacemaker response to sensing, programmability, and arrhythmia function.

Chapter 10

Get Moving

Now that I was awake, extubated, and had taken a quick assessment of what types of lines were coming out of my body, I should have a nice long rest to recover in the intensive care unit, right? That statement couldn't be farther from the truth. You will soon find yourself shifting to relieve pressure in different ways and determining how to best be comfortable in your bed. I would roll to one side trying to relieve some stress from my sore back muscles, but the new position would create pressure on my chest. I tossed and turned like the princess and the pea.

Eventually, you will find the position that works best to relieve pain and help you breathe the easiest that first day. Then a physical therapist will arrive and start talking to you about walking up and down the hall. Believe it or not, they aren't joking when they say it. My nurses were already discussing moving me and all the lines and bags over to the chair next to my bed so I could sit up on the first day. You have to get things moving. Move that fluid and move those lungs. You won't be able to pull yourself up with your arms, so you will have to rely on the nurses to come and get you transported to different places.

Trust me when I say you will want to get your body moving. Fluid retention is an uncomfortable situation you won't want to last. When you wake up from surgery your extremities might feel a little funny. You will most likely have a lot of extra fluid on your body and it could look like a balloon-sculpture version of yourself. Patients receive a lot of different types of fluids during the procedure and your body's natural balance gets shifted a bit while you are under anesthesia for surgery.

During surgery, your body is trying to compensate for what is happening to the changes in flow and pressure. At the same time, a perfusionist is trying to compensate for what is happening during the repair. And lastly, anesthesia is doing what is necessary to keep things in line while everything else is going on. It is a wild ride that you take your body for, and it will take some time for fluid levels to start diuresing and make you look less like the Michelin Man.

Diuresis is a process in which the kidneys filter superfluous bodily fluid. This process increases your urine production and the frequency with which you need to use the bathroom. If your body is trying to get rid of excess fluid, it would only make sense that if your kidneys work, that is where your system will default to push it out. Every milliliter of fluid that was put in your body during surgery was accounted for. That is why every drop of urine and glass of water is documented when you wake up. The goal is to try and re-establish your baseline levels of fluid without getting your electrolyte balance out of whack in the process.

I was one of the few patients actually in the hospital for surgery during the pandemic, so I was heavy on staff. That was a huge benefit for me because there was always someone around looking for something to do because they didn't have the normal load of patients to take care of. The downside for me was that there was always someone around looking for something to do! There is no rest for the wicked, or post-surgical heart patients. You have the rest of your life to nap, so you may as well get to rehabbing.

During this time, my family still wasn't going to be allowed in to see me. Not even my wife. She called the nurses' station a lot, which was understandable. After a day in the ICU, I had my cell phone so we could FaceTime. If you are ever curious about what loneliness feels like, having surgery where you can't even get out of bed on your own and then not being able to see your family for a week will clear it right up. And while this situation stunk for everyone involved, I was without my number one cheerleader by my side motivating me to push myself.

There were moments of feeling helpless, and that was scary. That fear can bring about some negative thinking that you will need to push out of your mind. I am sure a lot of patients will ask themselves why they had the surgery at all. The consideration that surgery was not worth it at this point is like looking at a fender bender and claiming you should have never driven in the first place. There is an entire life ahead of you once this repair is done. Listen to your family. Listen to your therapists. Get your ass out of bed and keep moving forward.

The facility where I had my surgery had a large staff of young nurses. Fast-paced, high-acuity ICUs have a siren call for aggressively goal-oriented nurses who like the challenge of a busy environment. For my stay, they happened to be all female. Not that I care one way or the other. I am just stating the facts.

The only reason I mention this is because of the graphic story I am about to tell you. Everyone that worked with me was extremely nice and very capable at their job. Despite believing they were all capable professionals, I still felt bad when I had to ask them for help with a slight problem I was encountering. It was a natural process. My bowels had returned to normal, and even though I hadn't eaten since the day before surgery, I could sense my body needing to have a bowel movement.

I was sitting in the chair next to the bed at the time. I pondered if this sensation was real, or the possibility that it was just gas creating pressure on my abdomen. Everyone's bowel habits are different, but I can go from a potential sensation to a prairie dog in a matter of minutes. As it turned out, this was not gas. In thirty seconds, my situation had evolved from leaning left to fart in my chair to clean-up in aisle three if we didn't do something immediately.

Here I sat, unsure of what needed to happen. I did know it would have to happen relatively soon. I waved my beautiful and innocent young nurse over and embarrassingly explained the situation. Obviously, she has done this many times before, so she didn't bat an eyelash. My nurse explained it was a simple process of helping me to my feet, placing a bedpan with a chuck under me, and letting me do my business. A chuck is nothing more than a thin disposable pad for beds. The plan did seem simple.

Do you want to know what wasn't simple? The process. My ribs hurt, my back hurt, and I wasn't supposed to be lifting myself on my own. So here I am, all six feet three inches and two hundred forty pounds of me. I am having a five-foot-nothing nurse that weighs a hundred pounds help me to my feet, lines and tubes flowing out of me connected to plastic containers on the floor and bags of fluid on IV poles on wheels. I looked like some dystopian fellow waking up from his pod in the Matrix.

My nurse made this event look effortless. I realized that adjusting lines and tubing while supporting my weight as she placed the bedpan was a process she had perfected over time. Here I was, sitting on a bedpan in an open view of anyone around in the unit, trying to pass a bowel python. It was a magical moment.

I kid you not. My body was telling me I was nowhere close to done, and I was running out of the bedpan. I had to motion my nurse back into the room mid-process. She then had to call a friend over to help me stand and support me so I could try and finish this disaster. If I was at home, I might have had to call for measurement for a world record.

But here I stood, a young female nurse on each arm, in terrible pain wondering if my intestines ran in a straight line for three feet. After it finally stopped, the poor girl had to take it away and clean my backside for me. I have often wondered if I was the reason that someone went home from a job they had loved and said, "It's over, I'm done." I spent a fair amount of time that day contemplating surviving heart surgery only to die of embarrassment in the ICU.

I do hope she stayed because everyone there was awesome. The physical therapists had me walking daily. My nurses made sure I was eating, and my pain was managed. A respiratory therapist came and walked me through the incentive spirometry so my lungs would expand appropriately. Even my anesthesiologist stopped by to check on me. Each and every person was professional and friendly about helping me with my postoperative recovery while in the ICU.

Looking at everything in hindsight, I believe having major surgery during a pandemic was a wonderful experience. Throughout your time in the hospital, you will be surrounded by individuals who did not happen into healthcare by accident. They are extremely well-trained and caring people who want to help others. They are so good at taking care of people, they don't even flinch when you are having one of the most embarrassing moments of your life.

An incentive spirometer is a device that measures how deeply you can inhale. It helps you take slow, deep breaths to expand and fill your lungs with air. This helps prevent lung problems, such as pneumonia. The incentive spirometer is made up of a breathing tube, an air chamber, and an indicator.

Chapter 11
The Cardiac Stepdown Unit

Once you have started making the appropriate progress in the cardiac intensive care unit, it will be time to free that bed up for the next patient. Your next destination will take you to another specialty care unit called the cardiac step-down unit. This unit will still have specialized nurses who are experienced in caring for cardiac postoperative patients. The monitoring will be a little less intrusive than it was in the cardiac intensive care unit. When it was time for me to be sent to the step-down unit, I still had the majority of the same intravenous lines in place. The exception was the arterial line that was used for my blood pressure. It had been removed before the trip to a new room.

I would only be having my blood pressure taken periodically at this point by a cuff pressure. As the appropriate checkboxes are being checked off, there isn't a need for minute-to-minute monitoring any longer. Once the chest tubes start to produce less fluid, they will be coming out as well. This is a process, and things will slowly happen over a few days. No one will walk in one day and start discontinuing everything all at once.

One chest tube might come out, and later the second chest tube could be removed with the pacer wires. The central line will need to be pulled at some point as well.

Eventually, every line you have in your body will be removed, and you can head back home. It's a tried and true formula. Don't be impatient. Also, don't be nervous if you think something is coming out and it seems like it is too soon. Lines aren't scheduled to be removed by a calendar day. These decisions will be made based on the necessity of the line, looking at your overall status as a patient. Once the chest tubes stop removing an adequate level of fluid, they will be discontinued as well. These things happen when it is appropriate, not when it is convenient.

Once you get to your new room in the step-down unit, you will be seeing less of the nurses. Staff will still stop by at regular intervals to check your vital signs, but it isn't as persistent as in the ICU. Plus, your diet will change from liquids to some solids and eventually progress to a cardiac diet. Anytime food is involved, that normally makes me happy. I still appreciate pie. My speedo doesn't appreciate it, but the little things in life can make all the difference.

Each step forward is a positive moment that you can share with your loved ones as they come and see you, encouraging you through the process of healing. I guess. I am only making assumptions because, at this point, no one was still allowed into the building to see me. But I was still happy to pass this progress on to my family during our facetime chats. Think of every line and monitor removed as a tiny milestone on your journey to recovery.

A Cardiac Diet, or a heart-healthy diet, has the main goal of reducing sodium and saturated and trans fat intake. This can help minimize the effects of your diet on your heart health. This is a diet where you will eat nutrient-dense foods, such as fruits and vegetables, whole grains, and lean poultry and fish.

During this stage, my wife was sending me pictures and videos of the kids. She would text me to see if I was awake, trying not to interrupt the healing process. She would even Facetime and try to seem cheerful, even though I knew she was scared to death not being able to see me and touch me. My wife knew that I was alive because she could talk to me, but how comforting is it if you can't put your hands on that person?

Their smell, their touch, and everything you take for granted on a daily basis at home is unattainable at that moment. It was the beginning of a long journey for me, but that was possibly the longest week of my wife's life. She was quarantined in a hotel room with our three kids while her husband had major surgery next door. She waited days to speak to me, only to see me pale with lines protruding from everywhere. It makes my heart hurt thinking about what she went through. I know this story focuses on the patient, but every family member is affected in a different way by this process. Remember that fact when you think someone is being too doting and treating you like a child.

I was meeting new people over the days in the step-down unit. There were people who were checking on my incentive spirometry and making sure I was keeping my lungs healthy. Dietitians who explained that the flavorless food was good for me if I could try to actually eat some of it. I was finally able to meet the nurse practitioner that worked for my surgeon. We had only spoken on the phone prior to my surgery. She asked me about my healing and checked my incisions and tubes. I was also told she was going to be my contact person later in the process with any questions or concerns. This nurse practitioner would be the one taking out my lines and chest tubes and then discharging me home when the time came. It would be an understatement for me to say that this woman wore a lot of hats. She was pleasant, intelligent, and efficient.

This is a good time to tell you that the nurse practitioner (NP) or physician's assistant (PA) you will most likely be seeing is an extremely knowledgeable person who is an invaluable asset to your surgeon. They work with and for your surgeon every single day. If you believe that the things that they tell you are not that important or that you need to hear them from the surgeon, I have some really bad news for you. You probably won't hear them from your surgeon.

Nurse practitioners and physician's assistants are advanced practice providers of healthcare, and it is because of the work they do that allows the surgeon to see as many patients as he or she does on a day-to-day basis. Are you curious about who it is that is talking to patients for preoperative scheduling, writing orders in the hospital, and answering questions after you get home? If healthcare is a machine, these people are the grease that keeps everything moving every day. So be respectful and definitely listen to what they tell you.

These advanced practice providers will be the ones writing your prescriptions for pain meds. When the hospital gives you postoperative care instructions with a number to call for questions, do you think a surgeon will pick up when the line rings? In reality, it will be one of these individuals who has spent years specializing in a discipline so you and I can see a surgeon in a reasonable amount of time. It will be the first time you have ever asked someone a lot of these questions. It will be the hundredth or thousandth time this practitioner has answered those questions.

My nurse practitioner is a lovely person. I had spoken to her over the phone several times and had a decent relationship with her coming into the surgery. The times that I saw her in the hospital, she was full of information. Yet the day she came into my room to remove chest tubes and pacer wires, it made me start to wonder if she had a side job as a dominatrix. I mentioned earlier that I had decided to take care of pain control with acetaminophen. This was one of the days I regretted that decision immensely.

My advice to you would be to ask the nurse for something for pain prior to chest tubes and pacer wires coming out. An anxiolytic would have been preferred for me, but an opioid might do the trick. Also, for the love of everything holy, look away while it is happening. I could care less watching an IV going into my body since I have placed thousands of them myself over my career. I assumed this scenario would be the same. I thought there might be a little pull and that would be it. Just for a recap, I'm an idiot.

The chest tubes and pacer wires do have to come out of your body. Those don't go home with you. The tubes are stitched into your skin, so they don't come out until the precise moment they are intended to do so. The day that this event was happening for me was exciting. This was another mini-milestone that I could tell my wife about later.

My nurse had mentioned that they like to time this event with some narcotics to make patients more comfortable. I am admitting this here and now so I can't claim later that she didn't give me a fair warning. My nurse practitioner assured me this was a fast process where a patient could take a deep breath, and once the stitches were cut, the chest tubes and wires would be removed. It all sounded so simple. Just a quick moment in time, and I was on to the next progress step.

This might make you nervous. It made me nervous. Because every time I had told a patient that propofol might sting a little, I knew in the back of my mind there was always the chance it might burn like acid in their vein. I took the assurances of my nurse practitioner with a grain of salt. I completely ignored the recommendation of the cardiac nurse for pain meds. I just sat in the bed, watching the whole process happen.

No medication was taken for this, just haphazardly believing that I had made it this far with only acetaminophen, so I should be fine. The nurse practitioner cut the stitches. A little pulling at the skin with some tweezers to make it easier to cut free. It pinched a bit, but that was easy. Stitches feel like a tickle to me when they come out of the skin. I thought to myself, this might be the worst part of it. Again, I am borderline delusional.

The nurse practitioner took a firm grip on the tubing and then smiled, looking me right in the eye. "Take a deep breath." Before that breath was fully in, she pulled the first tube in one swift motion from my chest. It wasn't painful, but it wasn't pleasant either. I tried to object, but there was no time. Her hand was already on the second tube! Instead of breathing in, I just tried to prepare myself, but it was too late. She was pulling the larger tube out now. What little breath I had was taken away by the sensation of chest tubing exiting my thoracic cavity through a hole cut below my sternum. I couldn't look away as she calmly extracted the tubing as casually as grabbing a snake by the tail in her garden.

As she talked about how easy that was, tying up the stitches that were left behind to close the incision, my mind was still processing the event. Imagine someone calmly telling you how solid the slap to the face had been while your cheek was still throbbing from the blow. It was surreal. This woman is a professional, and those holes where chest tubes had been were already closed up. She was smiling and working as I tried to take a moment to catch my breath.

I heard something about a little tug, and the next thing I knew, the wires that were clipped for security to my heart were yanked free and extracted as well. I would say this took my breath away, but I'm not certain I had taken a breath at this point. The whole ordeal took less than five minutes, and the pain was no more than a stubbed toe. Yet the rapid procession and casual tone still left me feeling a bit violated. Nonetheless, the tubes and wires were gone, and I was one step closer to being able to go home.

I would talk to the nurse practitioner several more times, explaining how things were healing, and hearing what I should expect next in the process. A flurry of individuals stopped by for different reasons during the next few days. Physical therapy is still getting you moving day to day. You will start this process with a walker and all the tubing hanging from it, and only a few days later, be walking slowly beside therapists under your own power.

Respiratory therapy is making sure you are breathing deeply to avoid any atelectasis, which is collapsed alveoli in the base of your lungs due to a lack of expansion. This can cause infections and prolong your stay with other problems, so listen up when the respiratory therapist is talking. You want to consistently be forcing air into the base of your lungs to push that fluid away and maintain a healthy lung capacity. No one ever tells the story of when they were in the hospital and got pneumonia due to fluid collecting in their lungs, and it helped them heal more quickly. Because it doesn't.

However, the best part of my stay was definitely my cardiac nurses. Again, my stay was different than most. The hospital was emptier than it had ever been, and nurses didn't have many patients, if any at all. My family wasn't allowed in the door, so I had no one coming in to cheer me up or check on me. There was only a phone to say hello to everyone in my family while they stayed quarantined in their hotel room.

My nurses played two roles for me. They managed my care and medications as well as anyone who has ever taken care of me in the past. Out of compassion, or perhaps boredom, the cardiac nurses would also come into the room and talk to me for extended periods. One shift would relay to the next what my job was and where I lived. The next nurse would come in and ask me about those things and keep my mind active about things other than the fact my family wasn't with me, and I had pain all over. Those nurses were not required to do that for me, but I will never forget it.

Something to keep in mind is that the people that take care of you when you are in the hospital are just like you when they aren't at work. Each and every provider has their own life, problems, and worries. Yet, they leave them at the door as best they can to take care of others and make them as comfortable as possible. For every person that can tell a story about some awful nurse being mean to them, I can tell you about a time I had to bite my tongue for a patient who was being unruly or rude.

These staff members can have bad days just like everyone else. I know that I can have bad days at work. I am sure that you do too. If you are the type of person who is, for lack of a better description, a festering irritation, your stay might not be as pleasant as it could have been. This is the staff that will monitor your health and give you medicine when you need it. They will bathe you and care for you when you cannot do it for yourself. In my case, this will be the group of people who keep me from wallowing in a vat of self-pity out of loneliness and boredom. The medical staff will be your personal guardian angels during your hospital stay. It only makes sense to treat them accordingly.

An important component of your healing process and your personal satisfaction is nutrition. I know I love to eat. My transition up the dietary chain was reasonably rapid. I was excited to hear that with each step, new items would be available for me to add to my diet. A lot of people complain about hospital food. At the time of my surgery, I have worked in numerous different hospital settings over the years. I have never found the food to be bad at all. I actually have fond memories of some of the meals served in the hospital cafeterias where I have worked.

That is not how this story is going to go. Perhaps my taste buds were off. Maybe the medication I had taken affected my appetite. Whatever the reason, the food in this place tasted like the south end of a skunk headed north. There were times my nurses and dietary staff had to force my hand for caloric requirements postoperatively. If you find yourself in the same scenario, I will encourage you to suffer through it and make sure you are eating enough food. You don't want to be any weaker than you already will be when it comes time for a walk up and down the hall.

Due to the pandemic, my surgeon did not want to waste any time getting me out of the hospital and back home. The normal process after discharge is to stay in town for three days for a quick follow-up with the nurse practitioner. I soon learned that an appointment was not going to be required. I should get home, and we could do the follow-up virtually. This pandemic was new to everyone, but I understood it was for my safety. Plus, I had many hours of riding in a car with a pillow strapped to my chest to protect me from the seatbelt to contend with. My team wanted me safely away from any place where contact with a virus would complicate my recovery. I did not need convincing. I was ready to see my family.

The last checkbox that had to be completed before discharge was imaging. This will involve another echocardiogram and a CTA. These imaging tests will be your new best friends after surgery. You will be sent back to the famous donut imaging machine to get everything from chamber dimensions to flows checked. This is the surgeon checking his homework before turning it in.

If you have a procedure like mine and paid attention to the numbers preoperatively, this is where you can find out how much work was done. My aneurysm was at 5.5 cm before I got on the table, and now it was sitting at a smooth 3 cm. My natural valve had been saved, so everything in my surgery had gone as planned. This sounded great at the time. Mission accomplished. If there are no complications and you have not had any issues during your stay, this is the time to pack your bag and put on your grippy-soled slippers.

This is also the time that one of your wonderful cardiac nurses will come in to talk to you about discharge instructions. These instructions can include who to call for problems, follow-up appointment dates, how to take your prescriptions and even rehabilitation. There is enough information to cover that you get a binder stocked full of reminders. You also might get a heart pillow, which I will touch on in the next chapter. Prescriptions can normally be filled as well for the trip home. Then everything is all tucked away into a carrying bag for your convenience.

All of this will be covered in a span of less than half an hour. You will probably be less than a week out of your surgery at this point. Please, pay attention here. Have a family member in the room to listen to these instructions with you. I was alone, and every time my wife asked me a question that I know was covered in the discharge instructions, I had no idea what the answer was. You won't be in Mensa form at this stage of the game. Your mind will be cloudy from surgery and drugs, so it will be a difficult scenario to retain information. Hence, the folder full of the answers to those questions that they packed for you.

My total time in the hospital was five days. You heard that correctly. From the time I showed up and was shaved chest to toe, had my ascending aorta replaced, and left the hospital was five days. 150 years ago during the Civil War, soldiers had amputations done with saws while they bit down on rags. Those soldiers had a total mortality rate from amputations of 26.3% according to Robert Reilly in his article *"Medical and surgical care during the American Civil War, 1861-1865."* That same article notes that another 45% of soldiers would die from post-surgical wound infections.

I just had a man cut my chest open, stop my heart, fix it, and send me home in under a week. This situation makes you take a moment to consider how productive you have been the past seven days. This is amazing stuff! Although this might all seem overwhelming and scary to you, these procedures are done every day and are remarkably safe for patients. You are ready for this, and so is your team.

Chapter 12
Let's Go Home

Now the day has finally arrived. It has probably only been a week, but time passes differently when you are recovering from major surgery. You are walking the halls, eating all your delicious meals, and your doctor says you are ready to head home. There will be moments while you are lying in your hospital bed when you will wonder if this day will ever come. When it finally arrives and you get your discharge instructions, you might start to get nervous about being at home without someone watching over you. The freedom you wanted can feel scary and overwhelming. It's like the first time your mother asks you to go get milk all alone after waiting for your driving license. The world suddenly seems bigger and faster than you have ever noticed it before.

These feelings are normal. As thoughts begin to swirl in your head about all the things that need to happen once you are home, do not stress yourself out too much. The majority of people have felt the same way that you might feel at this moment. You just need to understand that this journey can only be conquered one day at a time.

Go ahead and take the first step confidently. Of course, it will only be stepping into a wheelchair to get transported to the front door at this point. Someone might be holding you by the arm to steady you as well. Baby steps are still steps.

If you have to travel home in a vehicle for an extended duration, make sure you are taking regular breaks to get out of the car and walk around to minimize the risk of blood clots. Blood thinners are part of the medication regimen to minimize the normal risks of blood clots after surgery. Sitting for long periods and not generating blood flow to your lower extremities is a recipe for disaster. Frequent breaks are a good tip for any of you road warriors, but an especially important one if you are traveling by car after your open-heart surgery. I say "traveling" because you won't be allowed to drive for quite some time, depending on what your surgeon feels is appropriate. Also, consider sitting in the back seat away from the airbags and put a cushion or pillow under any seatbelt that crosses your incision. This is a great use of your heart pillow.

What in the blue blazes is a heart pillow anyway? I don't know if there is a technical name for it. I am sure it could be location-dependent, like johnnies and hospital gowns. They are the exact same thing but called something completely different in the north and the south. My heart pillow was also in the shape of a heart, so it was doubly correct in calling it as such. This pillow is a medium-sized, soft-to-the-touch, relatively firm addition to your recovery.

This pillow has a practical use aside from padding your incision from your seatbelt. You will keep this thing handy in the event you need to cough or sneeze after your surgery. You can squeeze the pillow nice and tight to try and minimize movement of the area around your incision and theoretically reduce the pain involved. That does not mean a hard cough will be pain-free. I am still wincing and having pain six months out from surgery when I have to sneeze. Some relief is better than no relief. And some cushion between your incision and the seatbelt in the event of a quick stop is better than none.

Once you are back at home, you will be free to just relax and kick back with no therapist bothering you and no nurses taking your blood pressure. Just kidding. If you were in the hospital for a week, and recovery is months and months long, the time at home is where the actual process of healing begins. There might not be people enforcing the therapies and breathing exercises, but that doesn't mean the therapies are over.

The hospital is the area where practitioners make sure you don't have any weird stuff pop up after surgery. Things like arrhythmias, lung issues, or bleeding. Home is where your body has to take the time to heal itself. In theory, home is the place that should be viewed as your sanctuary. Your home is the easiest place to relax in the comfort of familiarity. However, if you want to heal effectively, you will need to push yourself out of your comfort zone and get motivated. This is no vacation.

This is also the time that any normal person in a normal situation would talk to their surgeon about cardiac rehabilitation. Cardiac rehab is a great time to meet with other people who have had cardiac procedures and talk to them about what is happening in the healing process. You can even have therapists ensure you are moving enough and getting back to where you need to be from a cardiac standpoint. This place will be full of bikes and treadmills to get your body moving and on the road to recovery. There will be weights available once your sternum is healed to strengthen those atrophied muscles. Cardiac rehab is a conglomeration of work and motivation, shared by people who are working towards a common goal.

At least that is what I am told. Of course, cardiac rehab was shut down for the pandemic, so I was told to follow the instructions in my booklet and call with any questions. I can tell you right now, I had plenty of questions. However, I found myself questioning whether or not to call anyone with these queries. Some of my questions felt silly to ask. I felt unsure who was the best fit for the provider to take the call in my situation. My advice for dealing with this situation is to call anyone and everyone. Get the answer to your question twice if need be.

I didn't want to be a bother. Occasionally, I justified my defiant nature to call and ask for help by believing that because I worked in surgery, I should know these answers. Asking questions felt like an inadequacy in my career. Administering anesthesia in surgery and having surgery are two different worlds. I made a lot of mistakes postoperatively when it came to feeling comfortable asking for help. I am telling you about these mistakes so you don't have to make them.

When you ask questions about your recovery, you are not a bother. You are someone who needs information that you don't currently have. Your providers are trained to answer those questions. You should utilize their expertise. I get questions every day about any number of things related to surgery. I love answering those questions. But I still let a little pride get in the way of seeking help when I felt vulnerable. Trust your providers to be knowledgeable and empathetic. Be better than I was and swallow your pride if it gets in the way of your recovery.

All of my follow-up was being handled locally by a cardiac surgeon at the facility where I work. It was the same surgeon I had ambushed in the hallway with my results before this journey began. My surgeon in Ohio knew it wasn't reasonable to have someone going back and forth between states for every follow-up or question. The surgeon was several states away and his staff were available for my concerns, but it is easier if you are working with someone locally to field questions when you have them.

I went in to see my local cardiac surgeon after the first week I was home for my initial follow-up appointment. He pulled a few stitches for me from my drain site and checked things out. The surgeon checked my incision sites and listened to my heart and lungs. You want to check for healing, drainage, and red areas that could be irritated. Everything was looking good for me, so I was told to try and avoid the hospital during the pandemic if I could. This was definitely not the time to be getting exposed to any virus that I would need to be intubated for treatment. The lockdown was in full effect, so my journey to recovery would be lived out in solitary confinement at my house. Thank goodness my family was there to support me.

What should the focus be now that you are at home? One of the first things you need to do is define the best process for medication management. There will be a plethora of drugs on your daily regimen once you get out of the hospital. The medications can vary depending on the type of procedure you had and your surgeon's preferences. Since you aren't exactly in the prime of your life after surgery, this is the perfect time to have someone help you get organized. There will probably be some medications due once a day and others due twice a day. There will be bottles for breakthrough pain that need to be separated and labeled with something so they will stand out. The only difference in the look of the majority of these bottles will be the label. The tiny print that requires I find my bifocals is my only hint as to what I am holding in my hand. This is not ideal.

Daily pill dispensers, colored lids on pill bottles, or whatever it is that can keep things straight for you will work in this scenario. There will be some concoction of aspirin, multivitamins, beta-blockers, possibly an antiarrhythmic, and even a blood thinner. There will also be medicine available for normal pain relief. Then there is an additional bottle for above-normal pain, also known as breakthrough pain. That is a lot of different medications for a post-surgery foggy haze that you can find yourself in.

A good idea would be to keep the pain medication bottles separate from the others that are for daily use. Maybe even keep a notepad handy and write down dates and times when you take those pain medications. You can even make a journal to track what happens daily throughout your recovery. This could include pain, anxiety, dizzy spells, and what medicines have been taken at what time. If there is a problem that you don't need to deal with postoperatively, it is mixing up medicines or taking too much of something that could make you even drowsier or clumsier. Falls are a big negative right now. Protect yourself at all times.

With that protection, now is a good time to talk about fall-proofing your house before you get home all shuffling and frail. How easy is your house to get around? Do you have stairs you need to consider? Is there a multitude of throw rugs around your living spaces? What about floors that can be a little slippery like hardwood or tile? If you have ever had to childproof a house and learn a new system of precautions for a bit, then you can do this. Just imagine yourself as a clumsy child making their way around your current home, and your only job is to keep them safe.

This process can even go so far as lowering items you might need in a medicine cabinet to a point where you don't have to lift your arms above the designated degree that will be set by your surgeon. If it helps, imagine yourself as my wife sees me. Envision a guy who is so borderline incompetent that he can't move around or feed himself without guidance. I might be an idiot or a genius depending on how you look at it. Think through your daily routines. Find the tripping hazards and reaching scenarios that you can get rid of before you do something silly and hurt yourself.

Where do you sleep? That probably strikes you as a dumb question. Your rest will be of the utmost importance when you are trying to heal postoperatively. Because it will be beneficial in the healing process to be sleeping slightly upright while avoiding sleep on your side and stomach, a logical alternative is to sleep in a recliner. If you have a recliner, as many people do, then you are in a good spot. If you are like me, who has not had a recliner for many years, it might be time to go shopping. For all the men who love shopping as much as I do, this is not the time to utter the infamous line "just get me whatever."

My wife and I searched far and wide for the perfect chair to keep me comfortable and safe once I was home from surgery. I sat in chairs at every store in my area. We didn't want leather because it could be cold when I first sat down or stick to my skin if I got hot while I was sitting. I wanted it wide enough to accommodate the breadth of my ass, but not so wide that I had to bend over and reach for the pull handle to extend or retract the footrest. Well, why didn't I just get an automatic version where I could push a button and watch the footrest raise or lower? I looked at those too! I found these types of chairs less comfortable than the chair that I chose.

Ultimately, this is a personal choice about what feels best for you. You will more than likely spend a fair amount of time in it while healing. It would be nice if you will be able to rest comfortably as well. The chair might appear to be a silly thing and that any recliner will do. For every person thinking that right now, I want you to think about your shoes. How far are you willing to walk if your shoes don't feel comfortable? The same principle can be applied to your sleep and the comfort of your back. Many people have survived cardiac surgery without a recliner. This is not a must-have item. I am only mentioning that the recliner is a great addition to a positive recovery period if you can manage it.

Rest is an extremely important part of the recovery process. You want to be able to find a way to be safe and comfortable while you are on the road to recovery. Any chair or bed that adds to the amount of soreness your body has will only make it that much more difficult when it comes to moving around in a rehabilitation setting. The key to my rest was comfort and the ability to stand up without having to support my weight on my arms.

Lifting yourself up and putting stress on your pectoral muscles are a big negative after you get home from surgery. The stress on your pectoral muscles can also stress your incision site and the wires or bracket placed to keep things immobile. When I mention that you should make sure your toothpaste is at waist level, it should go without saying that lifting yourself out of a chair with your arms is a bad idea. But I will say it anyway. Do not use your arms to lift yourself out of a seated position once you get home.

An often overlooked component of recovery at home is if you have pets. We covered earlier that you needed to make arrangements for pets to be fed while you were away, but what happens when you come home? Currently, there are two wonderful Dalmatians in my household. Beautiful, high-energy, loving animals. Two of the descriptors that I just used can be a problem for a postoperative heart patient. Do you have small pets? Do you have multiple large pets? Do any of these pets tend to want to jump in your lap when you sit down? Do they like to be at your feet when you walk around the house?

You will need to make considerations for how those scenarios will be handled once you decide to grab a seat for some much-needed rest. I have one Dalmatian that weighs eighty-five pounds and believes he is a teacup Chihuahua that needs to be a lapdog at all times. If you are unexpectedly hit in the chest by a pet, a couple of things can happen. Most commonly, there will be a large helping of pain, served with a side of discontent. You won't need any additional measures of pain during the recovery process. You will have plenty to deal with without adding to the pile of symptoms.

Another problem that could occur is damage to the surgical site. If a pet trips you and you instinctively put your arms down to catch yourself, you could break some very important things loose inside your chest. If you add a broken bone on top of the rest of surgical recovery, you are stacking the deck against your success. So, you have to manage those pets. If it means room divider gates, crates, or sending them away for a bit, you need to do whatever it takes to keep yourself safe. Again, you are a clumsy child with poor balance and a propensity to hurt yourself if you fall.

The next thing you might want to consider doing or have someone else help you do once you are home is developing a schedule. Medications can make you drowsy, and healing can take a lot out of your energy level. These things can make you sleep more than usual. Recovery from cardiac surgery is not a television marathon, eating popcorn and sugary snacks until you are all healed. A daily schedule should include when you are headed to cardiac rehabilitation, your medications and when they need to be taken, and intermittent walks around the house to keep blood flowing and increase lung capacity. A schedule tells you what needs to be done. A journal tells you what has been done. It is a subtle difference, but an important one.

If you have a schedule made up and posted somewhere close by, it can make things simple to look over and stay on task. It will be even easier if you add a clock with large numbers close by. You will be able to see exactly what needs to be happening when you rub your eyes clear of crud after your third nap of the day. You can also add a checklist of healthy nutritional items and goals if you think that eating will be a challenge after surgery. Medications can affect your appetite. They can also dam you up like the Hoover. A schedule is a great way to steer activities in the direction of what needs to be done when you don't want to do any of them.

Exercise will be your best friend and your worst enemy at the same time during the recovery process. The more movement you initiate to keep your body systems flowing, the better your recovery will progress. Those same movements will hurt you physically and even mentally at times. It can be mentally taxing to know that a short walk exhausts you when you could stride out several miles before surgery. This is a temporary situation patients need to push through. Along with exercise, you can also incorporate snacks that might loosen up the works and keep you from having any intestinal issues. Who could have guessed that a healthy diet and exercise leading to a healthy body would still be accurate?

One of the things you shouldn't be doing postoperatively is straining. And what do you think you are doing if you are sitting on the toilet bearing down? Keeping yourself regular might seem like a no-brainer, but it can be a challenge when you are lethargic from medication. The last thing you need to do is hold your breath and try to push too hard on your thinking throne and pass out. It is much easier to eat prunes than have the emergency department sew up your head from a fall off the toilet. Remember the story about the guy that fell off his toilet and was knocked out, but when they found him a day later his heart was all healed up? Me neither.

The schedule will become important for everyone in the house. Depending on the situation you are in when you get home from surgery, some accommodations might have to be made for transportation. If your spouse has to go to work, and you have cardiac rehabilitation, how will you get there? If you have a follow-up appointment to check incisions, are you planning to walk to a bus stop since getting to the bathroom will probably wind you once you are home?

Perhaps you are making plans for recovery without considering the fact that you cannot drive when you get home. The length of time is dependent on the surgeon, but you can expect to not be behind the wheel for a month at a minimum. You shouldn't be raising your arms to the level of the steering wheel, twisting your body to look around, driving while on medication, or being that close to an airbag. You will need a ride, so the schedule comes in handy to determine when someone outside the house might need to be called to help with getting you where you need to be.

A quick checklist of things to consider after surgery...

- A medication management system
- Preparing the house for a postoperative patient
- A journal to keep track of activity and medication

- A schedule to keep you on track
- Regular movement and exercise
- Adequate rest

None of these items are required by any means. Some people might tell you they made it through with none of these things. Other people might tell you to add more things to this list to help once you are home. At least now you will have some ideas about how to prepare your home for your arrival back after surgery. Does this mean you now know everything you need to know about surgery? Perhaps, but more than likely not. This has been a bare-bones guide to the very basics of open-heart surgery. The next part of this guide is going to discuss in detail some of the things that you might not hear about at all before surgery. I certainly didn't hear about them.

Not all of these things will happen to everyone, but I will discuss my personal experience of what happened to my body after cardiac surgery. Read at your own risk. Just remember, it doesn't matter how scared you get at some of the possible side effects because the alternative to not having surgery is often death or, at a minimum, a diminished quality of life.

I know that might sound brutal, but we are talking honestly here. Read ahead if you want to know what some of the possibilities might be. If you don't want to know, skip it. Like your recliner, it's a personal choice. I am the type of person who would like to know what all the possible scenarios might be to mentally prepare for those things. I also don't want to wonder if I am crazy because something seems out of the ordinary. I feel better knowing crazy is just a part of who I am.

Chapter 13
This Wasn't In The Brochure

Now that your surgery is over, what should you expect from your body when you get home? This chapter will be dedicated to what happened to me personally. It will describe some of the surprises that awaited me once I got back home. Bluntly, this is a very descriptive retelling of all the things that I should have expected as possibilities during the recovery process.

However, I didn't expect them because quite a few of these things weren't truly in the brochure for the surgery. All of these items are only possibilities, some of them being only a minuscule chance. That is why most patients don't hear about them. There is a very high likelihood that many of these symptoms won't affect you. If they do, then this chapter is dedicated to your sanity.

Where do we possibly begin? The most obvious starting point when it comes to major surgery is pain. That is the number one thing people asked me about. Pain is what people will ask you about. Average greetings will change from "how are things" to "are you hurting"? People don't want to know the details of your surgery, but instead will ask you the level of pain your chest incision is giving you. It is an odd scenario I would liken to people wanting to put their hands on a pregnant woman's stomach. Thankfully, they won't be reaching toward your chest. It might be the wrong question, but people don't know what else to ask when pain is the biggest curiosity.

Instead of it being a complete mystery, let's discuss what you might be experiencing once you get home. While this chapter will describe what I felt, and remember that pain is a subjective state. Every person experiences pain differently. I was taught in school that pain is whatever a patient tells you it is. If your pain is less than my pain, that doesn't make me a liar. It only makes all of this even more confusing when trying to decipher what will happen to you and what is normal.

The area of concern for you and everyone else will be that big scar running vertically from the top of your chest down to your upper abdomen. The pain associated with the midline incision is not what I assumed it would be. Or maybe it was, but the additional accompanying pains overshadowed it for me. What did it feel like? A cut. A big-ass cut, but a cut nonetheless. It might be similar to the incision on a total knee arthroplasty without the joint soreness. I have never had my knees replaced though, so I am still only guessing. I had my foot sliced open and sewn up when I was younger, and my chest incision felt similar to that. But that probably doesn't help you much either.

Initially, it will be tender to the touch. Once the incision starts to heal, it might feel tight around the wound. You might notice the stages of healing running through the incision. While cleanliness and wound care are imperative, the majority of my discomfort came in the form of muscle pain.

Stages of wound healing from woundsource.com...

Hemostasis phase - This phase is characterized by blood flowing to the area of an incision. This stage will be cut a bit short by the use of cautery to stop the actual oozing of blood from the wound itself during surgery. Platelets will form to start the clotting process. Clotting will add fibrin, which works to bind areas together. After surgery, the sutures will accentuate the fibrins job by holding the incision immobile. This phase will happen while you are asleep in the operating room.

Inflammatory phase - Inflammation will begin soon after the initial incision occurs. The injured blood vessels will leak transudate, which is a substance made up of water, salt, and protein. This will cause inflammation, which is the body's natural defense against bleeding and infection. This swelling allows for healing and repair cells to move to the site of the incision. It also helps to remove bacteria and pathogens from the site. White blood cells, growth factors, nutrients, and enzymes are what cause the incision to appear warm and red. Warmth is normal for some time and is only problematic if the elevated temperature persists. This could be a sign that there is still bacteria in the incision.

Proliferative phase - This phase is characterized by the wound being rebuilt with new tissue composed of collagen and extracellular matrix. The incision will contract as the new tissue grows and develops. New blood vessels can be formed to bring oxygen and nutrients to the granulation tissue forming at the site. In the final stages of this phase, epithelial cells will begin to resurface the incision site.

Maturation phase - This can be known as the remodeling phase of the healing process. Collagen will remodel from type III to type I and the wound will be closed. It is the cross-linking of collagen on the incision that causes the thickness of the wound. Remodeling can begin about 21 days after the incision was made but could take a year or longer to complete.

When the chest spreader is placed in your thoracic cavity, the process of making room for the surgeon to operate and spreading your ribs apart at the sternum creates immense pressure on your back muscles closest to your spine. Imagine if you stretched your arms as wide and as far back as you can right now. Go ahead and try. The harder you reach behind your back, the tighter your muscles get. You can start to feel stress on those upper back muscles and tension toward the center of your back. Now imagine that your surgeon has just freed up the range of motion by cutting through your sternum and shoved those muscles even closer together.

Now that the muscles are bunched together like commuters in a rush-hour subway car, you get to keep those muscles in that position for a long period. This creates some very sore areas in your back. These muscles cannot be stretched out to relieve the pressure you are feeling once you are home. If your calf muscle is tight, you can put your toe on a step and stretch that tightness away. You have to remember, your arms have a limited range of motion when you get home. Stretching habits are out the window for the initial stages of the recovery process.

Positioning becomes a very uncomfortable thing after surgery because of these sore muscles that you have. Add on top of that an inability to move and stretch the way you normally would to relieve some of the tension. Now, I don't want you to think that muscle pain will be isolated to your back. Your pectoral muscles will get stretched and pushed back from your sternum as well. It is a combination of the front pectoral muscles with the back muscles that creates a sense of soreness and tightness in your chest that is difficult to work out.

This soreness can present a greater pain to contend with than the actual incision site. If you are in a car wreck and don't break any bones, no one assumes you just go home with no pain. Your entire body will feel the after-effects of the trauma. These manipulations and stressors on your body can be a significant factor in how the recovery process progresses. You will have to find a coping strategy that keeps you moving despite the soreness. Sore muscles do not go away with inactivity.

Imagine scenarios where activity isn't your go-to when working soreness out of a muscle. You might want to try heat applied to the area. You might want to try a light massage. What was my answer to sore muscles? Years ago, I had a back injury, and my wife found some small transcutaneous electrical nerve stimulation (TENS) units that can apply electrical shocks directly to areas of pain or tightness. I utilized those to flex and relax the muscles repeatedly until the muscle started to loosen. This is a situation where you have to find out what will work best for you. Think outside the box if you have to.

There won't be any long, hot baths for quite a while once you are home. You can't sit and soak a fresh incision site. Even if the site is healed, hot baths that vasodilate your blood vessels will lead to increased dizziness when you try to get up after you are done. You also won't be able to pull yourself up using your arms initially. All of these very basic methods have to be reconsidered with your body's limited ability after surgery. These weaknesses don't persist but can be prolonged if patients aren't careful with activity once they are home.

One of my greatest pains was associated with a relatively small area. When I say small, I mean the actual size of a large needle. The site where the central line was placed in my neck would remain sore for much longer than I anticipated. It is an insignificant incision compared to the one in your mid-chest area, but the area where it was placed was sensitive to the touch for considerably longer than most other incision sites for me. This soreness on my neck lasted for weeks. When I was brave enough to touch my midline incision, it didn't cause the wince I felt when I touched the dot incision from the central line. I wish I had an answer to why that was. Unfortunately, I do not. There is always the possibility that the line went through a muscle on the way in, but I can't say for certain.

South of your midline incision will be a couple of smaller incisions where the chest tubes and pacer wires were placed. These can be sensitive as well, as they both penetrated the thoracic cavity and will have stitches in place. These incisions are not normally as uniform as the straight chest incision. Where the midline incision has someone taking the time to sew it up as linearly as possible, the chest tube holes are tied up in a matter of moments.

The smaller incisions sit closer to the bend in your abdomen and can tend to be uneven or rough. This uneven texture can also lead to a collection of oil and dirt, so it will take extra care to keep them clean. The soreness will soon give way to itching with the stitches. Once the stitches come out, there will be scabbing. Try your best to avoid scratching at these areas. Cleanliness and self-restraint are the keys to effective healing when it comes to incisions after surgery. Don't pick at wounds or uncover them to check the progress.

While tender initially, these areas do not tend to be a source of great pain. If they become red and irritated, this could be a sign of an infection. An active infection will ramp up the pain level as well, and that would be something you need to talk to your provider about if it were to happen. Some antibiotics might be in order. But if kept clean, the chest tube incision site will not be a source of pain that keeps you up at night. If the pain is something that is bothering you, make sure you are taking your standard pain medications that were prescribed. There are no awards given out for people who can handle this situation without any pain medications.

This might be another great place to make notes in your journal as you evaluate your wounds. You can make notations on the size and shape of inflammation or feverish temperatures. If you are taking medications and get confused about the specifics of your wound healing, your notes might be just the bit of information you need to avoid a call to your doctor. The description could be as basic as 'the size of a quarter, thin red line surrounding it, itches like my foot fungus.' Keep it simple and relatable.

Like all incisions, especially large ones, there will be bruising. Some of the bruising can be attributed to anticoagulation therapy from surgery. Depending on your age and personal blood counts, there might be more bruising for some than others. The bigger the bruising, the more soreness you can encounter from that blood trapped in the skin.

As bruises age and change colors, it denotes the body's metabolizing of the byproducts of broken capillaries. The bruising will be ugly, but it shouldn't affect your day-to-day activity level or lack thereof. If you look down at other areas where lines were placed, you might see the same telltale sign that some bleeding occurred under the skin. Treatment for bruising might involve applying some heat or elevating the affected area to clear some of the trapped blood. Some people believe eating certain foods will accelerate bruise healing as well. Foods high in bromelain, like pineapple, have been mentioned in some literature to help speed the process. I didn't concern myself with my bruising. Without doing anything special to treat them myself, I can't speak to the efficacy of these natural modalities.

Now let's discuss your breathing. This is when you will be getting lectured about the incentive spirometry device to make sure you are taking plenty of deep breaths to expand your lungs. Do it! Breathing will be tricky with the soreness in your chest and back, but you have to keep filling the bases of your lungs with oxygen or you run the risk of getting fluid in there. There are a lot of ways to speed up recovery. Pneumonia is not one of them. That is more of a way to see how resilient you are if you are the kind of person that likes to tempt fate. I do not recommend trying that.

What area will hurt while you are blowing into that plastic tube of the incentive spirometry? Every muscle in your chest that we talked about earlier will make itself known as you exercise your lungs. These sore muscles will be pushed and pulled every time you take a breath. The point of incentive spirometry is to expand your lungs beyond the capacity of an average respiration.

Collapsed basilar alveoli are called atelectasis. You will be forcing air deep into your lung bases to change the pressure gradient and expanding those alveoli. This exercise increases the surface area in the base of your lungs to enhance oxygen exchange. This also means you are also stretching out those sore chest muscles beyond what a normal breath is as well. You will put pressure on the incision on your chest. You will pull at the incisions in your abdomen. This level of discomfort can make you want to minimize the actual size of the breath you take during the exercise. You have to move past that defense mechanism. So many times in life I have heard the phrase "listen to your body." When it comes to deep breathing, this will be one of the times you will have to ignore it.

I have found that whenever I take a deep breath, I can feel my heart beating in my throat. I don't mean a fleeting beat or two. If I hold my breath, I can count my heart rate as accurately as if I was taking a radial pulse. This isn't painful, but it gives you an eerie feeling that something might be wrong. You can feel your pulse in your ears when you deep breathe? Completely normal! There's a statement I never planned on making.

An important thing to note would be that your anatomy might not be identical to what it was preoperatively. Anatomy can get slightly moved around during this process. My chest expansion was uncomfortable to the point that the sensation of my heart beating in my throat affected me mentally as well as physically. On the physical aspect of deep breathing, I couldn't wear my CPAP at night initially. The filling of my lungs put immense pressure on my chest, and it felt as though my heart was going to beat out of my throat. It wasn't, but that was the level of the sensation for me. It took me a considerable amount of time to move past that feeling and put my CPAP back on to make sure my lungs were being expanded properly at night.

Another part of the healing process can involve orthostatic hypotension. This is basically when you rise from a sitting position to a standing position, your circulatory response is slowed, and you could feel light-headed and dizzy. The changes in blood pressure are regulated by baroreceptors in your carotid arteries and aortic arch. Theoretically, nothing has happened to these receptors during surgery. Yet, a common occurrence after being on bypass is dizziness associated with positional changes. This is especially dangerous immediately following surgery for several reasons. If you are dizzy and you fall, you could injure yourself. While bruises might seem bad at this point, the main focus should be on your unhealed sternum. I can assure you that once you have reached the point of getting back to your home in the process, no one wants to knock something loose and start over.

A second consideration is the fact that your natural response when you are falling, or even trying to steady yourself from dizziness, would be to put your arms down to catch yourself. This is another bad idea when you get home from surgery. It will be painful, and you run the risk of opening up incision sites or even breaking wires maintaining sternum stability.

If you are a heavier-weighted or stronger individual, your body and strength will supersede the tenacity of those wires that can be put in your chest. They will break, and then you have to head back to the operating room to have your wound opened again and those wires replaced. My surgeon determined that he didn't want to risk it, and the decision was made to use a plate on my sternum based on my age and stature. I am far from a superhero, but that is my point. An average individual can find themselves in a situation they do not want to revisit if they aren't careful.

What causes the dizziness or hypotension in this case? There are a few theories. You can take what your doctor tells you at face value, but the certainty of what causes it in each individual is no more certain than the severity of cases from one patient to the next. While one person might not experience this at all, another might find himself wavering months or even years after the surgery. There are averages, and there is your normal. Those two things might not be anywhere close to one another.

My personal experience has been dizziness with position changes for many months after surgery. These instances can vary in severity for me. It can cover a broad spectrum of symptoms from instance to instance. One episode I might feel a bit light-headed, and the next instance I might feel as though I am going to blackout. I can steady myself with one hand for one situation, but have had to lie on the floor for a half hour with another. Again, there is no normal. There is only your experience.

This is nothing to take lightly but also nothing that is concerning to the surgeon initially. I have even encountered some vertigo-like situations over the months following surgery where I couldn't stand up for a while. I just lay there and watched the world spin. It scared me enough to ask my local surgeon about it. My doctor was once again reassuring me that these things take time. Occasionally, more time than you think is normal. Your patience might be tested, but you can persevere through these nuisances.

Without the benefit of cardiac rehabilitation sessions, I found myself with no one to ask what was normal or abnormal with my recovery. After a few weeks of issues, I started to get concerned about some of the things that were happening to my body. I called my local cardiac surgeon's office and made an appointment. I did that even though he had said to stay away from the hospital to avoid the chance of Covid. That was how concerned I had become with these things happening to my body. The unknown was affecting my mental state of being. I needed answers.

Later the same afternoon, my phone rang and the cardiac surgeon was on the line. I am sure he had listened to the same false panic numerous times before. I am dizzy! That is normal. My chest still hurts! That is normal. I am having trouble remembering things! That is normal. My list seemed fairly insignificant after chatting with him. The surgeon was calm and collected, which helped me get calm and collected. Weird things that feel completely abnormal are exactly the norm in a lot of cases. That is why it is important to ask questions and find out what other people are experiencing. The mental stresses of feeling alone and isolated in what is happening to your body are an unnecessary burden in your recovery.

One of the theories you might hear about several of the side effects of heart surgery will be attributed to cardiovascular bypass. Again, this is the time in surgery the surgeon will refer to as being *on pump.* The details of that process were discussed earlier, but a quick recap is simply bypassing the circulation in your heart for the time in surgery it takes to do the repair. The cardiovascular bypass will be the time your body is subjected to non-pulsatile flow. This is a high stressor for your body.

Leaving some arteries with no flow for a time can lead to a loss of some vessel contractility. That same contractility is what can control blood flows that need to get to your brain in certain scenarios like standing from a sitting position. Less contractility means lower pressure and less ability to send blood flows as quickly as your brain might demand them. This isn't permanent but can take more time to heal than expected. You should allow an adequate amount of time to pass before concerning yourself with the question of if it is normal. I have been told numerous times this situation goes away. I am six months out, and the frequency of dizziness has diminished for me, but not gone away. I am acutely aware, but try not to be concerned. There is a difference.

An additional side effect of bypass surgery that is not mentioned very often, because why scare you if they don't have to, is a phenomenon called pump head syndrome. I don't mention it now to scare you. I am telling you because when you haven't heard of it and it happens to you, it can be far scarier than if you had been able to prepare for it. This is a scenario of the devil you know being less intimidating. If we discuss it now, there could be less panic later.

Pump head syndrome is a post-perfusion scenario that isn't defined as an actual syndrome, but more of a collection of neurological symptoms that can occur for some people after they have been on bypass during surgery. When you hear medical terms like postoperative cognitive dysfunction, you might discern that they are saying that your pump head could make you feel like an early-stage dementia patient. It certainly sounds severe. How concerned should you be that this new memory loss will make you unable to return to normal? The answer is not concerned at all.

This event can be scary, but it is extremely rare to persist. I remember getting a concussion in my junior year of high school in a football game that landed me in the emergency room. The situation of recognizing people around me and not knowing anyone's name was unnerving. Imagine a thought that is on the tip of your tongue that you just can't verbalize. While losing your train of thought mid-sentence is frightening, it is not something that is concerning initially following surgery.

Even months after the fact, some people can find it persists in a small manner. People might tell you that you have already asked a question that was answered and you might not remember it. You might have an entire conversation and lose it. If it is any consolation, I remembered all of my children's birthdays, just not what I had for lunch the day before when I got home from surgery. This will clear up over time. Cautionary family members might panic and think you are having a stroke. You are not, so let this be a reassurance to them. Maybe that will avoid an expensive trip to the emergency room.

The important thing to know is that pump head can happen. It isn't necessarily a permanent condition of the surgery. An even more important thing than the condition itself is to discuss this possibility of it happening with those that will be spending time with you after surgery. This is so they don't get concerned or frustrated with the scenario. When you are already scared that something might be wrong, it does not help the situation to have someone laugh or get angry about something you won't even understand is happening.

Most people probably just read that and thought to themselves, "Who would laugh at someone having problems with their memory after heart surgery?" I can think of some people. The good news, I do still love them, and none of them were kicked out of the house. The old saying that laughter is the best medicine is not accurate with heart conditions. You need surgery. However, aside from the soreness in my muscles, I did find laughing a positive aspect of my recovery process. Being angry or bitter won't speed anything up. You may as well have a laugh, even if it is at your own expense.

The next topic is something that can happen in a small percentage of heart surgery patients.

Depending on who you ask or what study you read, the actual occurrence rate can vary a great deal. When I asked about this problem with my first call of concerns, I was told that some degree of this situation could occur in up to forty percent of patients. I then read a paper where the occurrence rate for the study was four out of seven hundred patients. As I discuss it, take this with a grain of salt. We are only talking about possibilities, no matter how insignificant.

What is this thing that can happen? Visual disturbances or visual changes can occur after surgery as well. Here is where people are very divided on what that means to them personally. Some people might believe that their eyesight sucked anyway, so what will a small change mean to them daily? Probably not much. However, this scenario can be as varied as the occurrence results.

Some patients might find that they cannot discern any visual changes at all that have occurred. One day you find yourself at the eye doctor getting your annual checkup, and they mention that you have had a slight deterioration in your eyes and need a bump up in your prescription. This happens with normal aging, so a person might not even associate it with their surgery. We will use this as an ideal situation in this context.

Others might find that they noticed a vision change and went in and needed more than a bump up. This patient might have gone in because they noticed that even with their glasses on, the words on the page were still hard to see. Occasionally, there can be a higher degradation of vision that occurs in some patients. Either way, if you are one of these people, get a new prescription and move on. This is one of the side effects where things probably won't be passing and returning to normal. Your new vision after surgery will be your new vision from now on. I am in my mid-forties and have to wear bifocals. Does that suck at a young age? Yes, but at least I can still read with them on. All things become a matter of perspective.

There is a tiny chance of another scenario that can occur as well. This is a more concerning type of visual disturbance to the patient, but still not something that the surgeon would get worried about initially. While both of my eyes did degrade after surgery, requiring a new prescription, I also found that on occasion, my eyes would start to have some wavy flashes around the peripheral edges. These waves slowly creep in until my vision is more of a small tunnel directly in front of me, with the remainder being wavy flashes of light that disrupt my field of view.

My vision loss would last anywhere from half an hour to an hour normally. Over time, the occurrence rate will theoretically drop. There are no specific things that caused it for me that might be attributed to circulatory changes like rising from a sitting position. Some activities that require physical exertion might bring it on. Other times, physical activity does nothing.

The scariest thing about this situation is that no one could tell me how or why this was occurring. No one could tell me if it was going to stop either. Initially, several times a week at an arbitrary time of my eyes' choosing, my vision is diminished to nothing more than if I was looking through a paper towel tube. It was not painful or associated with any other side effects like headaches or migraines. I just sat and watched the sides close in on me until the majority of my vision was gone. As with most things, patience is your friend. I didn't have any patience, but I am asking you to be better than me.

There is a minuscule chance that you could have visual disturbances too. While this provides you with the perfect opportunity to panic, I hope that you can remember this moment and relax. It won't make your vision any better, but it can avoid the awkward scenario of telling your spouse you might be having a stroke and need to go to the hospital. The only things you will find there are frustration and a huge bill.

My personal experience was visual episodes that had progressively gotten worse to the extent of happening several times a week with no answers in sight. I was stressed about this scenario, and I saw many smart people trying to figure it out. Many possibilities were explored, but time was the only answer. It isn't scientific, but some weird things happen to your body that people will try to rationalize for you. Occasionally at the end of the day, a provider can just say, "I have no idea what that is."

Even before I even had a solution, I would tell you that this situation is better than waiting around to have my aneurysm dissect and possibly kill me. No fear or irritating side effect is greater than your need to fix what is broken in your heart. If this happens to occur, take a seat and relax. I tell myself it is my body's way of telling me to slow down. Forget about the limitations of your body before surgery. There will be an entirely new set of rules postoperatively that you will learn as you go when it comes to activity.

The biggest issues we have discussed postoperatively involve pain, soreness, bruising, memory loss, and a tiny possibility of vision loss. All of these things can happen in varying degrees, or possibly not at all. There could be a huge list of other issues tackled here as well. The main point of this section was to give you an idea that many different scenarios could occur, so you don't think you are crazy if it happens to you. Talk openly with your providers and other patients at cardiac rehabilitation about what is happening to your body.

Some people have more difficult recoveries than others. I just want you to remember that even the weirdest side effect can be nothing at all. I remember waking up in the cardiac ICU and looking down and seeing my penis was purple. I lamented to my wife it might never work again. She laughed, I cried. I like to think it was because she knew I was overreacting, not because she thought of the minutes it would save her in the bedroom. Recoveries are intimately personal, but you should still feel comfortable asking others if they experienced anything similar. Well, maybe keep your penis problems to yourself.

I am not saying you should ignore problems or not ask your provider if you have questions. Just try to remember that abnormalities are completely normal! You can do this. If you are here mentally preparing for the challenges that might lie in front of you, you are already well beyond where I was when I started this journey. A positive state of mind and a strong support

network are the keys to getting through this with
your sanity.

Chapter 14
Should I Be Concerned

As you have read through this information, a common theme might have started to emerge: Should I be concerned about all of this? Absolutely! And, no. This is a plethora of information that is being given to you so you can start mentally preparing for surgery. There are some checklists you can use to expedite your planning phase. Take a minute, a couple of deep breaths, and try not to get overwhelmed by all of this.

But how can I not be concerned? After everything you have heard about what can happen, remember that there is a chance that nothing will happen as well. Pain could be less than anticipated, you could have 20/20 vision, and you could be back to your normal routine in no time. That isn't the most likely scenario, but still a possibility. If you are concerned about some of the less than ideal things that can occur postoperatively, I want you to remember this tip that a doctor friend of mine gave me when I was complaining about my frustrations in dealing with all of these things during recovery.

You didn't die...

That is number one on every checklist that you can put together for surgery. No one who heads into the operating room to have open heart surgery is there by accident. I have yet to talk to a single patient who was on their way to the grocery store and took a wrong turn into the hospital and was admitted for surgery. Something in your body was broken to the point that it could have affected your quality of life or even your longevity of life. These plans are now being made to give you something that you would not have otherwise. You are getting time. When your eyes flutter open, and you hurt, tubes and lines protruding from everywhere, remember that this is temporary. It is the beginning of a journey to better heart health. It is also the hope for a better quality of life.

If you are reading this quick take on your heart surgery, then you have already begun to prepare mentally for the path that lies in front of you. Many obstacles will stand in your way when it comes to mental preparedness. Fear, anger, and frustration might all rear their ugly heads at one time or another throughout the process. A positive state of mind will be your best ally in coping with what is going to happen to your body.

How do you stay positive in this situation? I am not a shrink that can steer you in the direction of coping mechanisms and the mentality to overcome whatever it is that affects you. I can only offer kind words and personal reflection in your time of stress. Try to imagine how you or someone you know dealt with the stages of grief in the past. If you have made it to this point in your life and can't imagine a time when you thought the stages of grief applied to you, then stop your worrying right there. You have lived a charmed life and have nothing to worry about now!

The five stages of grief are denial, anger, bargaining, depression, and acceptance. If you deny you have a heart condition, you probably haven't read this book. If you had some health issues and went to a doctor who said you need open heart surgery and don't believe he is being honest, my best bet is you didn't look for ways to start planning. The denial folks are not here. But that doesn't mean it was a phase we got to skip in the process.

This stage might be best defined as the denial that I had in the beginning when I kept pretending my chest pain was nothing. Then when I saw the imaging results, I doubted that they would lead to surgery. I would encourage you to listen to your body. No one else can feel what you feel. They can help determine what it means when you tell them, but you are the only one experiencing it. No one can do this for you, and no one can help you if you don't ask for it.

Next, listen to the advice that medical professionals are giving you and take a moment to process them. Never be afraid of the question, "what does that mean?" No one in health care expects you to know everything that they are talking about. Ask the questions, pause for a moment, and absorb what you hear. Hypothetically, this stage has come and gone at this point as things have progressed to the point you are making plans. That means you are already making progress, and you haven't even had surgery yet. How awesome is that?

Perhaps the next stage that arrives is the time to get angry. Maybe you are the type of person that screams "why me!" You pound on your chest and lament the peril that has come to your life. But for all the rest of the people coping with a new diagnosis that this doesn't encapsulate, you should still have concerns about how you can handle this stage. Anger might manifest itself in comments to friends and family. You might be upset with things your spouse is doing during this process and not know why. Anger can control you without you realizing you have allowed it to manifest inside you. It can permeate conversations, subtle actions, and even the relationships closest to you.

This is one of the times when communication and the bonds you have built with those closest to you become the backbone of how successful your recovery will be. You can yell, cry, or just feel frustrated with those in the house that are not having to deal with what you are dealing with. It is the open communication and understanding that needs to happen to help build upon the supportive foundation you already have in place. Do not suffer in silence.

Let your family and friends know that you love them and cherish their support. You might even mention that there is a strong chance that you could become unreasonable and an ass at times. Let them know that it is part of the process and you will still need them when you are done being mean. Anger can make you verbally push people, just be careful not to push them away. If you feel like you have already done a fine job at building a wall between you and the people in your household, there is no time like the present to take it down and start mending emotional wounds.

The bargaining aspect will probably be between you and a higher power. Your surgeon might be open to some bargaining. He might be willing to deal with you on whether you have the first or second surgery of the day. You can find yourself in a position to bargain some meals out of your spouse if they don't want sushi and you do. Remember, even a small victory is still a win.

This is the perfect time in the process where those with faith might find themselves questioning, and then reinstating their belief system as a whole. In the United States, the Pew Research Center approximates 70.6% of the American population identifies themselves as being religious in one context or another. Whether you pray on your knees or talk on the treadmill, feel free to ask for guidance on the topic of clarity and perspective while dealing with surgery. Your personal deity might be God, Buddha, or Mohammed. Whoever it is you find solace with in a time of need, this is when that relationship will be explored more than likely. On that topic, I have a quick story to share.

I grew up in southeastern Oklahoma. This particular location is part of what most people would refer to as the Bible Belt of America. When people in my life started to find out that I was going to have surgery, I was added to prayer lists far and wide. They prayed in Oklahoma, where I grew up and where my in-laws still live. They prayed in North Carolina, where my mother is currently located. You might be aware of individuals who earn the moniker "prayer warriors." I had many prayer warriors adding my situation to their daily prayers. Big groups and small groups, all mentioning me by name for a smooth process and healing hands to guide me throughout.

But I also had someone else who had taken my cause to a higher power for me. A saintly woman who only knew me by chance for the last ten years, and who took my blessing to a completely new level. She carried her infectious smile with her everywhere she went. Anyone who spoke with her knew she was genuine and kind. This woman had never even met me in person, but she loved me. She was the mother of one of my family's dearest friends. He is like a son to me. And in her eyes, I was like a son to her.

This woman had trekked up mountains in China to Buddhist temples years earlier in her quest for faith. She might have been small in stature, but there was nothing that could keep her from the miles of steps required to see her faith reach its goal. Logically, when I needed support from a higher power, my own personal angel, Maxie, was on top of it. She had a Tibetan dZi bead sent to her so that she could take it to her temple and have it blessed. Once it was blessed, she asked if I would wear it throughout my ordeal. This blessed soul then proceeded to walk to her temple, light incense, and pray for me every day.

This routine continued for months. Rain or shine, Maxie would make the walk to the temple to light incense and pray. This became more than a routine. This process had transformed into another quest of faith on my behalf.

The entire time these daily vigils were happening, this beautiful woman, who had lost her husband the preceding year, was dealing with a personal ordeal of formidable magnitude. Maxie had been diagnosed with terminal cancer. A woman I had never met, who only knew me through her son's eyes and a couple of phone calls through the years, thought only of blessing me in her greatest time of fear and turmoil. The strength of Maxie to focus on the healing of someone else when she knew her personal situation was unalterable is still overwhelming to me.

After her passing, her son was at the temple for a ceremony celebrating his mother's life, and a monk pulled him aside to ask him a very important question that had been on their minds. Did he have any news on how my recovery was going? The monks had seen this beautiful soul pray over me so often, even they were vested in my recovery. That is a testament to Maxie's tenacity and faith in the most trying of times. This is exactly the type of angel you need in your life. Whether you believe in the power of prayer or the positivity of the universe, no one can deny the existence of something greater than themselves when faced with the love that Maxie showed me.

While you are bargaining your way through surgery, maybe you can make a promise to be that type of angel for someone else. There are few things in life that can bring more joy to your heart than feeling pure love. Whether it be family, friends, or a complete stranger, you will be overwhelmed when someone helps you without asking. I would only suggest that you do the same for someone else in return. We all have the power to change someone's life. The only thing stopping us is our own selfish interests. Be whoever you like in public, but be someone's angel in private. I promise you will never regret it.

The next stage is depression, which might be characterized during this time as fear or hopelessness. It can be easy to feel overwhelmed that everything that is happening to you is out of your control. You are relying solely on the expertise of others, which you have no concept of how someone even acquires in most cases.

I will ask you to recall the last time you stopped your car and turned around because you weren't positive about how reliable a bridge builder was at his job. Unless you have gephyrophobia, that number is probably zero. This is a time to try and cast fear aside and trust the capable hands of the team that is taking care of you through your journey. Just keep asking questions and communicating with those around you. This phase will subside, and you will move on to the acceptance phase.

Never allow this phase to keep you from planning and preparing for what is to come next. Do not let depression or fear drive a wedge between your support network. If a chain is only as strong as its weakest link, then don't get this close and let fear be the link that breaks you. Our lives are full of fearful firsts: first step, first jump in the pool, first kiss. Each and every one is terrifying in the moment, but fondly remembered as a pivotal part of who you are. This surgery is the same thing. A scary first that sets you moving into a new life. All you have to do is keep moving forward.

Here we are. I have finished my surgical journey, and perhaps yours is just beginning. I hope that this book might have helped explain some things, or at a minimum made you smile at my expense. The time is now to plan what you can, love who you can, and accept it all as nothing more than a small bump in the road on the way to a healthier life. If you have taken anything away from reading this, I hope it is to not stress over the things you cannot change and keep an open line of communication with every person involved. The people in your life love you and support you.

Occasionally, they might need a little guidance on the best way to do that. I hope that you are more prepared at this point to share with them how you can all move forward together in planning and preparing for your big day. There are lists to make and furniture to rearrange. You can do this! All you need at this point is to take it one day at a time. Keep putting one foot in front of the other, and this will be over faster than you can imagine. Good luck to you.

Two things define you: your patience when you have nothing and your attitude when you have everything....